# Dancing with Parkinson's

# Dancing with Parkinson's

Sara Houston

**intellect** Bristol, UK / Chicago, USA

First published in the UK in 2019 by
Intellect, The Mill, Parnall Road, Fishponds, Bristol, BS16 3JG, UK

First published in the USA in 2019 by
Intellect, The University of Chicago Press, 1427 E. 60th Street,
Chicago, IL 60637, USA

A catalogue record for this book is available from the
British Library.

Copy-editor: MPS Technologies
Cover designer: Aleksandra Szumlas
Production managers: Emma Berrill and Katie Evans
Typesetting: Contentra Technologies

Print ISBN: 978-1-78938-120-7
ePDF ISBN: 978-1-78938-122-1
ePUB ISBN: 978-1-78938-121-4

Printed and bound by Hobbs, United Kingdom.

To Fleur and Walter,
who encouraged me to follow
my passion for dance

# Contents

# Acknowledgements

My thanks first go to English National Ballet for believing in the research and supporting me to work with them for several years. I would particularly like to thank Fleur Derbyshire-Fox and her engagement team, and Tamara Rojo, artistic director, for making the research for this book possible. I also would like to thank English National Ballet, Rachel Cherry and Dance for PD for kindly donating the book's beautiful photographs.

I received financial support by way of BUPA Foundation prize money, which enabled the research to continue beyond a year and thence to a book. I took two sabbaticals to work on the manuscript and I am grateful to University of Roehampton for giving me the time to work solely on writing, as well as to the National Teaching Fellowship Scheme, whose prize money enabled me to extend my leave. I also benefited from a writing residency with Operaestate and CDC in Bassano del Grappa and my thanks go to Roberto Casarotto for his generous invitation. Thank you also to the Rayne Foundation and Dance Umbrella for supporting a visit to Dance for PD in New York.

This book was created following a long research process, through which a superb team accompanied me. Importantly, I would like to thank Ashley McGill, my co-investigator, who has been with me every step of the way through the process of research, analysis and discussion, and who made an essential contribution to the shape of the wider research – and also to the rest of the team, Raymond Lee, Katherine Watkins, Cameron Donald and Miranda Olsen. You provided wisdom, rigour, humour and constant support. I would also like to thank Brown University, Rachel Balaban and Julie Strandberg for supporting Donald and Olsen's internships with me.

I am grateful to all the dancers from all the dance for Parkinson's groups I studied, who gave up their time to speak to me and enthusiastically shared their thoughts, feelings and details of their lives, and a few their poetry, with me. You taught me much of what I know about Parkinson's. Without you this book would never have happened and you were the primary inspiration. Particularly, I would like to mention the English National Ballet London group with whom I danced weekly for four years and who embraced me as part of their community. Thank you to all who danced there for making the research such a fun and rich process.

There were notable others who gave up their time to talk to me and had the courage to let me observe them. In particular, the London and Oxford English National Ballet Dance for Parkinson's artistic teams, Danielle Teale, Rebecca Trevitt, Nathan Tinker, Jon Petter,

Nia Williams and Katherine Hartley were wonderfully accommodating and also were really open to furthering thinking together about dance for people with Parkinson's. Thank you for letting me hang out with you for so long. Thank you also to the volunteers and company dancers who spoke to me at English National Ballet and shared their thoughts, as well as to the artistic teams in Ipswich, Cardiff and Liverpool. David Leventhal at Dance for PD generously gave his time to discuss dance for Parkinson's and share information on many occasions. Thank you for your unequivocal generosity and openness. Your encouragement too was most welcome. Similarly those involved in the early days of the Dance for Parkinson's Partnership UK (the Network) welcomed me and have been fantastic in supporting my quest to understand the field. Thank you to you all for believing in my vision and allowing me to talk to you and observe your classes. There were a number of you who enthusiastically opened your doors to me and continue to do so in increasing numbers, so it is difficult to name everyone in person, but if you are reading this and recognize yourself here, this thank you is for you. I'd like to thank Kiki Gale and Toby Beazley especially for making me (and the book) feel a part of the Partnership. Additionally, thank you to the great many dance teaching artists, leaders and choreographers around the globe who did the same; in particular, Marc Vlemmix, Monica Gillette, Josef Makert, Pamela Quinn, Erica Jeffrey, Jane MacDonald, Olie Westheimer, Roberta Risch, Alex Tressor, Rachel Balaban, Andrew Greenwood, Vonita Singh, Hrishikesh Pawar, Hugo Tham, Clint Lutes, Gary Joplin, Giovanna Garzotto, Yasmeen Godder, Ofir Yudilevitch, Roberto Casarotto and Dario Tortorelli. The many conversations I have had with you have nurtured and fed into my thinking, inspiring me to probe the field further. I would also like to thank the Parkinson's activists and researchers who gave up their time to talk to me. I am greatly indebted to you for helping me understand this field.

A special thanks goes to Chris Jones, who was marvellously rigorous and patient in copy-editing the whole manuscript and who helped me set up the research website. You've seen the book and research in all its states of readiness and it would have been much poorer without your feedback and suggestions. Likewise, thank you to Stephanie Jordan, Anna Pakes, Annabel Stanger, Hakan Redjep, Theresa Buckland, Rachel Rakotonirina and Daniel Burges, who read and commented on drafts of the manuscript on top of their busy schedules. I am grateful also to all the help and support Intellect Books has given to first the idea and then to the realization of the book, and to the insightful comments given in the peer review process.

I am also indebted to my long-time mentor and colleague, Andrée Grau, who died as I was finishing the manuscript. Her passion for seeing the interest and importance in even small movements and the value in highlighting the dance of marginalized people has lived with me in the writing of this book.

I was kept sane during the writing period by going back to dancing myself after seven years of absence, which has in itself been a joy. The experience has fed into my thinking and writing, particularly the regular dialogue with my ballet teacher Brian Loftus. The writing process was also eased by regular trips around my local London cafés with my laptop. Lastly, thank you to Dan, Cameron and Ruaridh for your loving tolerance in putting up with my absences whilst I researched the field and wrote the book.

# Introduction

A clock is ticking and a heart is beating. Two adult men, one older than the other – mid-60s and mid-30s – stand in the light. They wear blue vests and shorts. They stand next to each other. The younger man casually lays his arm on the other's shoulder, his hand dangling down. They look at each other in the eyes and whilst they look, the younger, slighter man lifts up his companion's top with that hand. Meanwhile, he lifts his free hand up and wide and hits the older man on his bare stomach. The assaulted man proceeds to smack the younger across the cheek and takes him in a head lock. The younger retaliates by taking his father's finger and bending it back. He cries 'stop'. The father pinches his son's nose until his son pleads him to let go. The son attempts to put his finger up his father's nose. This fight continues, retaliation after retaliation; an arm is bent behind the back, nipples are pinched, fingers are bitten, ears are pulled. As the energy abates, the son lies outstretched on his stomach. His father stands balancing on his child's back, stretching out his arms to the side, as if he is flying.

Later on, the dancers' movements become tender, more caring. They carefully wrap around each other, their bodies melding into a ball; two arms unfold from this ball to mimic the flight of a swan, an echo of the earlier motif. And limbs interweave, one carrying the other. This care translates to a passage of movement where the younger man keeps falling over, his feet curling up, muscles spasming. His father tries to straighten his legs, but without success. In the final sequence the son climbs onto his father's shoulders and then drops down to his arms. Jimmy Fontana sings *Il Mondo* whilst the son narrates the story of their lives well into the future, when he is old and in a care home dying peacefully in his father's arms.

(Houston field notes on *Parkin'Son*, The Place, D'Anna 2014)

*P*arkin'Son (first performed in 2011 for Roma Equilibrio, Italy) was created by the choreographer Giulio D'Anna and performed by himself and Stefano D'Anna, his real father and an untrained dancer. It is a funny, emotionally turbulent, irreverent and moving dance work about the relationship between fathers and sons, about history and blood ties. What becomes clear within the performance, through the narration and in a moving solo by Giulio D'Anna, is that this work is influenced by, and in part about, his father's Parkinson's.

Father and son performed *Parkin'Son* 100 times during a tour around Europe. The physicality of the work is astonishing. At one point, the older dancer runs with his trousers around his ankles, catches his grown son in his arms, wrestles him to the floor and fights him. The risky interaction between the two dancers can be breathtaking. It is astonishing also because people with Parkinson's are rarely portrayed in such a physical light. In the extract above, no allowance is given for the pain or for the physical violence sustained or dealt out. Stefano D'Anna is not given any sentimental pampering or pity because he has a movement disorder that can leave a person physically and mentally vulnerable, and in return, he does not give any to his son.

Although as an artwork *Parkin'Son* is much more than a straightforward commentary on Parkinson's, it illustrates how dance can be a vivid way to illuminate the experience of Parkinson's. As an artistic medium that often uses movement to explore the embodied landscape of the senses and emotions, dance is well suited to highlight the experience of a condition, a neurodegenerative disorder, which often scars physically and emotionally. Thus, as a critically acclaimed work in a public arena *Parkin'Son* also documents and highlights the capabilities and humanity of people with Parkinson's.

This book, *Dancing with Parkinson's,* aims to explore the two avenues emphasized in D'Anna's work: how dance may explore or highlight the Parkinsonian condition and how the humanity of the Parkinson's dancers may shine through creative practice. More precisely, it demonstrates how people live with the condition of Parkinson's through their engagement with dance. In sum, it investigates the intersection between dancing movement, living with Parkinson's and the people who dance. The book argues that dancing enables people with Parkinson's to think differently about their condition in relation to their changing bodies. It contends that dancing can contribute to living well with Parkinson's and that this is partly to do with dance's aesthetic nature: art is crucial to the beneficial process.

The book was born out of a long-running research project at the University of Roehampton (Roehampton Dance 2010), led by myself, which began as a simple evaluation of a community dance group in London, United Kingdom. Little did I realize at the time of accepting the research commission that involvement in this project would become the basis for more than six years' investigation of an international phenomenon and would take me on a journey to several different countries. English National Ballet, a large-scale touring ballet company, ran the dance group and continues to do so. In line with many UK arts organizations in receipt of public funding, it has a remit to create outreach programmes, projects and events for community groups, the general public and for those who may not otherwise engage with theatre performances. Yet I quickly learned that this project with a group of untrained adult dancers was not just another education initiative led by a well-established dance company. The participants, dance teaching artists and musicians involved in the project were highly invested and passionate about keeping the weekly dance sessions going. The project struck an emotional chord for everyone in the studio. It reached beyond learning 'to do the moves', beyond just having fun. Dancing was somehow important. The dance sessions carried such significance for participants, notably, because they had Parkinson's.

Parkinson's is a neurodegenerative condition that usually develops after the age of 50.[1] It strikes primarily at the person's ability to move. As a practice that encourages participants to consciously think through pathways and challenges to moving in particular and various ways, notably in the company of others, dancing is well placed to address some of the issues associated with movement in Parkinson's. This book discusses this curiously well-matched – and exuberant – relationship between dancing and Parkinson's. It is concerned with exploring experiences of dancing and the activity's physical, social and emotional value for people living with the condition. *Dancing with Parkinson's* starts from the premise that the search for value begins by examining the points of view of the dance participants themselves, radiating out to look at their lives in context. It is a position that takes note of the subjectivities and individual circumstances of people living with Parkinson's in order to understand better the worth of dancing for these individuals. Understanding the value of dancing for people living with Parkinson's is the book's third aim.

As part of this investigation into its value, *Dancing with Parkinson's* documents the early growth of dance provision globally for people living with the condition. Although such documentation, by its very nature, will be overtaken by events and developments in provision, it stands as a case study of the emergence of a specialist area of community dance practice. It gives examples (but by no means total coverage) of different dance and teaching practices that have characterized dance for Parkinson's internationally in the first fifteen years of growth. The descriptions of various dance classes prompt a deeper exploration of dance movement in relation to Parkinson's in the second half of the book.

The speed at which dance provision – classes, programmes, performing initiatives, artist residencies – has expanded indicates the excitement and passion around the idea that movement may be of benefit to people with Parkinson's. Excitement generates many advocates and with this has come a small international community of scholars interested in studying objectively the relationship between dance and Parkinson's. Measuring physiological changes before and after dancing, the research studies have tried to explain, in concrete terms, the benefit of dancing.

Most medical research into Parkinson's is geared to help in finding a cure, or at least to understand the disease in more depth. In particular, scientists in the fields of neurology, biomechanics and pharmacological development have seen the importance of examining the condition. For a long time it was thought that exercise would exacerbate symptoms, and therefore, hardly any research was carried out on the effects of exercise on Parkinson's (Hirsch et al. 2008). Consensus has altered, and most neurologists recommend exercise to maintain health (see, for example, Hill 2009; Nieuwboer 2009). A growing body of bio-mechanical and neurological research is examining the effects of specific exercise, as well as ways to optimize motor control. It is through rehabilitative medicine that researchers became interested in dance for Parkinson's as a field of study. The majority of studies are focused on specific results from measuring balance and functional mobility where dance is a tool for a greater good, rather than something to be studied in its own right.

My own viewpoint as a researcher has been to argue for the importance of examining the dance itself, and dance for Parkinson's from a variety of angles. The book reflects this by building on the premise that dance is a complex social and cultural phenomenon. It can be conceived of as an artistic and creative activity, as well as a form of exercise and, sometimes, as a therapy. As a social activity, how it is used, presented, thought about and theorized carries political ramifications. The book emphasizes dance for Parkinson's as a social and artistic phenomenon, differentiating itself from the majority of research studies in the field that focus on it as a therapy.

I wrote part of this introduction in the corner of a studio bathed in sunlight in Bassano del Grappa, a city in the north of Italy. Whilst I wrote, Dario Tortorelli, an Italian dance artist and choreographer, described an improvised movement task to ten adults. There were many ideas from the group on ways to use the sunglasses littering the wooden floor as props. They were rehearsing for a performance taking place in an old church, now a theatre space, as part of the contemporary arts festival Operaestate. Three of the dancers had Parkinson's, each with differing qualities of movement developed by their symptoms. Later in the month, more dancers joined them for a week-long residency in the nearby mountains, working with dance artists to explore movement in a natural environment. They then worked up their findings into a more structured performance. The next year, the Italian dance artist Giorgia Nardin worked with four women aged between 45 and 80 from Bassano del Grappa; the eldest and youngest had Parkinson's. The show, *Stabat Mater*,[2] was premiered at the Operaestate Festival in 2016 and was a comment on womanhood, subversion and conformity. The power of the work came from the strength and maturity of the performers. The three residencies described here were offered as opportunities for the local community to create art through movement. They are illustrations of how dancing with Parkinson's is not a straightforward therapeutic activity to help with balance and stability. These examples, along with others where the work clearly has an artistic focus, have fed my conviction that dancing may offer people with Parkinson's much more than a physical workout and that it is possible to think of dancing as more than just a non-pharmacological medicine to alter disease symptoms. *Dancing with Parkinson's* explores the realm of dancing as an artistic and social activity, examining what its broader value might be.

*Dancing with Parkinson's* does not primarily investigate dance as an instrumental tool to overcome symptoms because dancing as art practice takes the participant on a journey that has no direct route to physical reintegration. There are not necessarily clear cause and effects that point directly to healing or management of illness. Unlike physical therapy practices, such as physiotherapy, dance as art refuses to create standardized, goal-orientated content that might be boxed and certified as clinically effective, despite the fact that some dance practices might be characterized as therapeutic. Art is not straightforward because it abstracts from the literal; it does not tell us stories and ideas in a literal way and so in creating its narratives, it often resists clear-cut conclusions. It prefers to provoke questions instead of answers. It involves flights of imagination. Its rules and way of doing things do not stand still but develop – sometimes radically, sometimes subtly – in the hands of different artists and participants. It is about stories, multiple interpretations and relationships. It is a practice that primarily provokes our senses, and which may or may not be translatable into words.

With these characteristics in mind, applied theatre scholar James Thompson (2009) argues that 'affect', not 'effect', is the powerful outcome within participatory arts practices.

It is limiting to think merely of the effects from participating. He writes: 'The impact of the work of participatory theatre cannot be distilled to the messages, story content or words, but must be opened up to the sustenance of sensation and the subsequent fuelling of inquiry' (Thompson 2009: 125). In creating a case for affect as the important outcome, he suggests that, stimulated by art, affect has implications for shifting perspectives and creating an environment where social change may happen: 'In this register, the effects are not foretold, but the affects stimulate – and being overcome by joy [...] or dancing [...] might loosen the icy grip of certain oppressive visions of how we should be in the world' (Thompson 2009: 125). The sensations experienced through the process of participating open out the way people may engage with others and with the situation in which they find themselves. Thompson proposes that for those caught in circumstances, such as war or ill health, which seem to impose certain ways of being, affects from participating in an artistic practice may plunge them into another perspective on their situation. *Dancing with Parkinson's* explores this opening out of positions, attitudes and bodily demeanours encouraged by participation in dancing.

Arts practices develop places of creative ambiguity where participants meet others, enjoy a conversation, laugh, cry, joke, swap stories, take on challenges, respond to provocations, relax, learn, create, fall in love, feel joy. In the dance for Parkinson's sessions that are described here, the people who take part are never called, or treated as, 'patients', and symptoms of Parkinson's are not the focus. In recognition of the art practices that lie at the heart of this book, and indeed of the qualitative methodology that characterized a significant section of the initial research study, the approach taken here is to focus on the person with the condition, rather than the disease as a biomedical entity. It is to emphasize dancing as a therapeutic pastime that is enjoyed by the moving person, rather than dancing as a tool to mend the sick body.

Inspired by the people living with Parkinson's who dance and create movement, and by those who facilitate engagement, *Dancing with Parkinson's* explores benefit through aesthetic values, seen from the point of view of the participant dancer and his or her engagement with dance as part of a group. So, although it does discuss some research studies that point to the influence of dance on the disease, *Dancing with Parkinson's* places the emphasis on the dancers themselves and their experience. Specifically, the focus is channelled into how participants articulate their dancing experience through aesthetic values, which *they* feel are important. Exploring aesthetic value, as Colette Conroy (2015) argues, allows us to explore the direct experience of human beings: 'Aesthetics enables us to activate analysis of the experience itself, to think in terms of our visceral and sensory responses and to extrapolate these into understandings of human agency and experience' (Conroy 2015: 2). Highlighting aesthetic values allows for the exploration of how, as human beings, we bring meaning into our lives.

Discussing aesthetic value develops understanding about why people choose to dance, what it is that makes dance as an art form different (or not) from other forms of exercise, therapy or art, and what it is about dance in its creative, artistic form that supports therapeutic outcomes. Moreover, investigating dance through examining aesthetic values within the participant experience exposes wider issues concerning construction of identity and how to live in the face of a chronic and progressive condition.

The book argues that the benefits of participatory dance for people with Parkinson's are understood best by examining the art form in relation to people's experiences, lives, needs and challenges. It illustrates this argument through studying several groups of people living with Parkinson's who have chosen to dance. It uses more than four years' worth of detailed qualitative data from the British Dance for Parkinson's programme run by English National Ballet, as well as six years of fieldwork related to other initiatives around the world, to ground the argument in practice.

This is an academic book. It adheres to the convention of grounding the argument through not only primary research, but also through the literature within relevant disciplines. The research follows in a sparsely researched area of qualitative scholarship investigating the phenomenon of Parkinson's. Two influential natural science projects of the nineteenth century first classified Parkinson's through observational studies of people with the 'shaking palsy': James Parkinson (1817) studied these people in an everyday environment, while Jean-Marie Charcot (1892) observed them within the confines of the Salpêtrière hospital in Paris. One of the best-known observational studies of the late twentieth century is neurologist Oliver Sacks' biographical account of Parkinsonian patients, published in his book *Awakenings* ([1973] 1990). Sacks studied a group of post-encephalitic patients in a hospital for the chronically ill, who displayed an extreme form of Parkinsonian behaviour. His work is particularly interesting because of his analysis of both movement and participation in the arts by his usually catatonic patients. In 2009, Samantha Solimeo published a large ethnographic study on people living with Parkinson's in Iowa, United States. Solimeo details the experience of life for her subjects and their carers, framed by a discussion of perceptions of ageing by those with the condition. Both Solimeo and Sacks' accounts bring to the fore what it is like to live with Parkinsonian symptoms, documenting the experiences, thoughts, feelings and emotions of those affected, as well as observations on the physical conditions of their subjects.

Likewise, *Dancing with Parkinson's* builds its argument partly using personal narratives of participants. It intertwines these stories with the social and political contexts in which the dancers live in order to examine the systemic and personal issues, attitudes and identities that colour their experiences of dancing. In other words, it weaves personal stories into an exploration of lives shaped by Parkinson's and attitudes inspired by dancing.

The personal narratives structure takes inspiration particularly from the work of sociologist Arthur Frank, whose ideas span the sociology both of the body and of narrative medicine. His work is interesting to explore in this context because he uses his own experience of chronic illness to argue for the need to tell and witness stories through the wounded body; to give voice to experiences 'that medicine cannot describe' (Frank 2013: 18). Frank argues that ill people have conceptions of how they should behave, which they feel are thrust upon them. He propounds that it is important for those people to create their own new ways of talking about their condition and of being themselves, thus giving voice to their experiences and conceptions of themselves with illness. These stories demand to be listened to and witnessed. They are coloured by 'different imaginations of illness', and Frank argues that 'these affect who ill people feel enabled to become' (Frank 2013: 187).

Frank describes some of these 'imaginations of illness' in detail, as individuals with chronic illnesses experience and narrate them. He categorizes these as stories or testimonies. He examines three narratives that are found within many people's individual stories, which tell of their hope to get better (restitution narrative), or of how they have decided to explore how they can live well with their condition (quest narrative). He also examines the state where people cannot yet articulate their stories because their world has been turned upside down with their diagnosis (chaos narrative). Yet for Frank, coming to a point where one can communicate one's own story and acknowledge that others may have stories that resonate with one's own is important in order to start to live well with illness.

There are clear parallels to the situation for the participants in dance for Parkinson's classes. The embodied nature of telling stories through dancing (whether these be structured or informal) allows participants to engage in communication with others. Their experiences of living with Parkinson's are told not just in speech, but also through their own movement. These experiences are rarely part of medical consultations or Parkinson's research studies; yet they are important to the dancers themselves, as well as to family members and the dance teaching artists and musicians involved. The resonances are strong between Frank's desire for people with chronic conditions to be visible and not ignored and how participants within the dance groups articulate a desire for dance to be part of their lives.

Frank is clear that a person's body and movement are central to telling illness stories and for *Dancing with Parkinson's*, this line of thought is crucial. Gay Morris points out that it is the task of dance scholars 'to look into how, where, and under what conditions the moving body is perceived in particular ways' (Morris 2009: 94). Yet the discipline of dance studies has not analysed in any detail the interesting equation of dancing and neurological conditions, leaving this to colleagues in dance movement psychotherapy, physical therapy and biomechanics. This arguably has to do with the newness of specialist dance practice in the area of neurological disorders and the tendency for both dance studies and dance science scholars to analyse professional performance, dance forms or cultures that include dance, rather than focus on populations whose bodies and movement are influenced by the symptoms of disease or syndromes.[3] This book addresses the gap in dance studies scholarship examining the peculiarities of Parkinson's, movement and the people living with the neurological condition who dance.

Exceptions to this are publications focusing on disability arts and dance, such as Fox and Macpherson (2015), Kuppers (2011), Henderson and Ostrander (2010), Benjamin (2002) and Cooper Albright (1997), although none of these works specifically mention dancers with Parkinson's. While people with Parkinson's would not necessarily call themselves disabled or ill, many deal with symptoms that threaten to curtail their active lives, many deal with pain and many fear encroaching disability (Solimeo 2009). Thus, the Parkinson's context has both affinities with disability arts and differences. Many case studies in the literature focus on congenital or static conditions, neither of which mirror the Parkinson's context, where disability may fluctuate and where the condition often develops after decades of neurotypical body function. Many case studies also deal with younger dancers and those who create art to celebrate disability, neither of which are usual situations for those with Parkinson's, as it tends to affect older people who want to be cured of the condition. Yet this body of literature addresses the question of who may dance and highlights what disabled people bring to dance. The works open out the landscape of dance scholarship to include those with atypical movement, and those with intellectual or physical impairment. In doing so, the literature brings to dance studies analysis of issues concerning social and cultural exclusion, movement form and function, and methods of teaching and art-making, among others. The politics of who dances and how are a clear theme within this literature and in *Dancing with Parkinson's*, albeit with a focus on a specific condition.

Most disability dance scholars propound the social model of disability to argue the case for inclusion. Early scholars and champions of the disability movement in the United Kingdom, such as Michael Oliver and Vic Finkelstein in the 1980s and 1990s, argued passionately and persuasively that it is the exclusionary behaviour of society that impairs and holds back disabled people, rather than the physical or mental impairments themselves (see, for example, Oliver 1990). This social model of disability has become mainstream discourse within disability scholarship and advocacy. Although *Dancing with Parkinson's* takes this line, it also engages with the experience of being impaired.[4] Disability scholar Carol Thomas argues that the social model has ironed out any argument about impairment. She notes that from the social model perspective,

> any focus on impairment or 'the body' conceded ground to the biological reductionism that had been orchestrated and sustained by doctors and other health and social care professionals for more than two centuries, a reductionism that lives on in discourses and practices in all social institutions.
>
> (Thomas 2007: 121)

In other words, the social model has refused to examine the material experience of being impaired as this might lead to accusations that impairments are disabling, rather than social barriers. Yet, as Bill Hughes and Kevin Paterson (1997) comment, it is incorrect to leave pain and impairment solely to medical science discourse. There are many 'personal and cultural narratives that help to constitute its [impairment's] meaning' (Hughes and Paterson 1997: 335), which disability studies – and dance studies – are equipped to analyse outside the methodological frameworks supplied by medical research. As Frank (2013) points out, the relationship of the body to medicine is limited by its focus on getting better, while the relationship of the body to its *experience* of illness and movement opens out the topic of impairment and pain.

It is worth highlighting at this point that in order to talk of the experience of dancing, particularly with a disability, it is not sufficient to talk of an individual's body, rather than of that person. It is not merely the body that experiences disability or dancing, but the person. This angle is different from other models of examining a person with a disease. Indeed, Hughes and Paterson see synergies between the medical and social models of disability's perceptions of the body: 'both treat it as a pre-social, inert, physical object, as discrete, palpable and separate from the self' (Hughes and Paterson 1997: 329). In dealing with the 'dynamic, living, presence of the body in movement and stillness' and with 'body relationalities' (Thomas 2003: 215), one is commenting on *people* moving.

Parkinson's is a condition that gradually reveals itself through various corporeal shifts of being, often with negative consequences for perceptions of self-identity. Turner writes that 'the relationship between my sense of myself, my awareness of the integrity of my body and experience of illness [is] not simply an attack on my instrumental body (*Körper*) but [is] a radical intrusion into my embodied self' (Turner 1992: 167). As such, Parkinson's lends itself to being studied as an embodied phenomenon. The participant-dancer's experience of moving enables me to uncover individual embodied responses to dancing and living with Parkinson's. Dancing offers an avenue for participants to articulate their experiences and ways of being through movement, as well as speech. Taking this into account, the book's focus is not on whether participants can be cured, but on highlighting people's relationship with Parkinson's whilst dancing, as well as on the modifications of their attitudes to moving and to living with Parkinson's. As there is no cure to date, people have to search for ways to manage and live well with their condition.

The primary source material used here comes mainly from multiple one-to-one interviews, focus groups, discussion groups, participant diaries, informal conversations and my observations from attending the Dance for Parkinson's programme led by English National Ballet over the course of four years. My original evaluation conducted for the company, mentioned above, was the starting point for further long-term research with the programme, with ethical clearance granted by the University of Roehampton Ethics Committee. The primary location for the dance sessions was the English National Ballet's headquarters in London. The programme subsequently established sessions in Oxford, Liverpool, Ipswich and Cardiff, cities to which the company toured. Data was gathered over a period of four months at each of these 'hubs' in addition to four years' worth of fieldwork with the class in London. In addition, I conducted interviews, together with observation and discussion, with teaching artists and participants in many other groups around the United Kingdom, as well as in Australia, Canada, Germany, India, Israel, Italy, the Netherlands, the United Arab Emirates and the United States. Many of these groups I was able to visit on several occasions, establishing lasting relationships with group leaders and participants. Their voices, poetry, ideas and movement are documented within this book and give a sense of the variety of approaches to dancing as well as exhibiting the sense of common purpose.

Interviews and focus groups were semi-structured, allowing interviewees to talk at will and go off the topic, which was useful in providing detail that may not have come up in a more formal style of questioning. Many people were interviewed several times – at the dance studio, in their own homes or at another location of their choice. Additionally, diaries, which were written in a variety of ways and in many styles, were windows to thoughts and activities that were often not aired face-to-face. Themes occurring within the data were identified and used as the basis for further questioning and conversations. Discussion groups were instituted to help explore these themes in depth. A group of up to eight volunteers were charged with discussing one particular theme. Sometimes they were also shown film footage of previous sessions to stimulate comment. Several of the themes identified are laid out as the primary topics of the chapters here.

The dance participants themselves were between 60 and 85. With a few notable exceptions, they were primarily at the first, second or third stage of disease progression,[5] although over the course of working with them, several developed more serious symptoms and three began the programme as wheelchair users.[6] All were welcome to take part in the ethnographic research and I am appreciative of the participants' enthusiasm to talk to me over a number of years, giving their time freely and with written consent.[7]

The two research studies conducted at English National Ballet were not solo efforts and included biomechanical and clinical measurement techniques to address some of the questions other researchers had been asking about physiological change. I include some of this work here, and I am indebted to my colleagues Ashley McGill, Raymond Lee, Katherine Watkins, Cameron Donald and Miranda Olson for their work in these areas (and to Brown University for supporting scholars Donald and Olson to work with me as research assistants). Their insights and work on the project have enabled me to examine the participant experience with a greater sense of the materiality of the body and its fluctuating physiological challenges, as well as the social and political issues that marked the experiences of the dance participants.

The book is divided into eight chapters and two parts. Part 1, comprising three chapters, describes the conditions that bring dance and people with Parkinson's together. It situates Dance for Parkinson's as a specialist community dance practice, placing it firmly within an arts, rather than therapy, setting. Chapter 1 sets the scene, describing the Parkinsonian condition in relation to how it affects people physically, socially and emotionally. Chapter 2 gives an account of the Dance for Parkinson's global movement, detailing classes, the approaches to facilitation and the teaching philosophies of its leaders. By no means exhaustive, the mapping of the practice worldwide does, however, give a sense of the early days of dance for Parkinson's work and the struggle to create a sustainable future. Following on from this focus on the teaching, Chapter 3 discusses what motivates people to dance and why dance specifically resonates so strongly with the Parkinson's community.

Part 2, through five chapters, explores the value of dancing for people with Parkinson's as expressed through the notion of living well with Parkinson's. The thrust of the argument is that the way dancing can affect participants aids their ability to maintain or develop a good quality of life. Each chapter examines one particular way that people claim to be affected by dancing. These 'affects' are translated as aesthetic values, namely, beauty (feeling lovely), grace (obtaining physical flow and dignity, receiving a gift) and freedom (forgetting about Parkinson's, obtaining movement control and valuing movement disorder). Each chapter develops by examining why particular participants hold onto the value in question within their stories of dancing and within stories of their lives. In doing so, the book argues for a re-examination of these age-old values, to look at them differently, from the point of view of participating in community dance practice, rather than as a spectator, and to articulate what these values actually mean in the context of people dancing with a specific chronic health condition. Rather than taking a mainstream contemporary view of seeing these values as superficial, apolitical or even disenfranchising (in the case of beauty and grace), the book argues for their importance to those who are attempting to enhance increasingly circumscribed lives.

Opening Part 2, Chapter 4 sets up the argument for an examination of values in connection to the benefit of dance for Parkinson's, rather than keeping the study within a clinical framework. The next four chapters focus on one value each. Chapter 5 examines the case of a participant who insists that the way dancing makes her feel lovely again is the most important reason to dance. It discusses why this feeling is so strong and how beauty can be valued within community dance, despite its intellectual marginalization. Chapter 6 examines several claims by participants that dancing makes them feel graceful, an unusual feeling for those with Parkinson's. The chapter separates grace into three categories to account for these claims: how a re-embodiment of flow takes place whilst dancing, how dancing can promote a sense of dignity and how dance encourages the sharing of different ways of thinking about Parkinson's through the idea of gift.

Chapter 7 explores the claim that dancing with Parkinson's generates a feeling of freedom. Freedom is described as 'leaving Parkinson's at the door', of not dwelling on the disease, which has a tendency to dominate everyday life. The chapter discusses the characteristics of freedom as they appear in dancing with Parkinson's: by embracing disorder, lack of control and risk as dancers, and, conversely, by the unusual opportunity to control and order the body whilst dancing. Chapter 8 highlights examples where communal motivation to dance has encouraged a strong sense of social bonding, reaching beyond the confines of the dance studio, and has aided participants in developing personal agency. The chapter puts forward an interpretation of agency and social action for those who live lives constrained by ill health and suggests how dance is a fertile environment to produce this amongst healthy and frail people with Parkinson's.

*Dancing with Parkinson's* is aimed at academics. It also will be relevant to postgraduate and undergraduate students with an interest in dance, Parkinson's, the arts and health, medical humanities, arts therapy and applied theatre. Without wishing to excuse the academic character of the book – it is important for dance studies scholarship that such a book exists in order to further conceptual thinking and to establish community dance as a serious practice to study – I hope that it also has relevance more broadly to those living with Parkinson's, to caregivers, to arts professionals and to professionals in health-related fields. It is possible to read this book as a case study in community dance practice, without any knowledge or experience of Parkinson's. Not many dancers with Parkinson's perform for a living, unlike Stefano D'Anna, who came to professional performance as a non-trained dancer, although several teach dance. *Dancing with Parkinson's* highlights the community dancer: those who fit in a dance class between going to the supermarket and making dinner, those who dance because they find pleasure and joy in moving. As Sue C (2013) comments in her diary: 'And you all make it such fun, so merry, there is such a lot of laugher'. But the mundane, the everyday-ness, in this particular community dance practice is hardly ever banal, as Josephine DG realized:

> I feel I have come so far since I first walked into the studio and wondered who all the people were on the far side of the room, not realising there was a mirror, and it was just us. I had no idea how dancing […] would transform my life.
>
> (Josephine DG 2013)

In the dance studio community art is precious, sometimes even life changing.

## Notes

1   One in twenty people with Parkinson's develops the condition earlier than the age of 50.

2   Nardin's *Stabat Mater* was one of four commissioned works premiered at Operaestate in 2016 with the same title. Yasmeen Godder, one of the other choreographers, also used local community participants in her work.

3   Both Manning (2009) and Soriano and Batson (2011) mention movement and Parkinson's within dance scholarship, and some of my work on the Parkinson's study has been published within the discipline of dance studies (Houston 2011, 2014, 2015).

4   This discussion was first aired in *Dance Research*, Edinburgh University Press (Houston 2011) and some of it is reproduced here.

5   The Hoehn and Yahr scale (1967) characterized five stages of disease progression and has been used widely by the medical and scientific communities.

6   Most had idiopathic Parkinson's, with a few suspecting they had a genetic form, and two had been diagnosed with an atypical Parkinsonism. Most people living with Parkinson's have idiopathic Parkinson's, where the cause is unknown. Approximately 5 per cent of people with Parkinson's have inherited it from a family member. There are other forms of Parkinsonisms, such as muscular system atrophy and progressive supranuclear palsy, which have many of the same symptoms but do not respond as well to Parkinson's medication. Some people develop Parkinson's due to a stroke or other head trauma, or through the use of certain drugs.

7   The Parkinson's dancers who volunteered to be interviewed, to write a diary or to take part in a discussion group wanted to be referred to by their real names in publications of the research. All interviewees were given the option of remaining anonymous and it is a testimony to how strongly they felt about others hearing their stories that nearly all elected to be known by their own names. In order to provide some sense of privacy on a personal subject I reference them by their first name and then, if they gave their last name, by the initial of their surname. (Some therefore are referred to only by their first name.) This referencing method also aligns with that used by other researchers, such as Oliver Sacks in his book *Awakenings* ([1973] 1990). When referring to Parkinson's dancers who have published their writing, I have used their full name because it is publicly available.

**Part 1**

Positioning dance with Parkinson's

# Chapter 1

Parkinson's pathology in a social context

## The shaking palsy

Although documents mentioning Parkinsonian behaviour date back to ancient Egypt (Palfreman 2015), James Parkinson, a doctor working in London in the early nineteenth century, is credited with the first detailed observations of the symptoms of the disease. He defined it as:

> Shaking palsy. (paralysis agitans.)
> Involuntary tremulous motion, with lessened muscular power, in parts not in action, even when supported; with a propensity to bend the trunk forward, and to pass from a walking to a running pace.
>
> (Parkinson 1817: 1)

Parkinson wrote this description in 1817 after extensive observation of six people with 'the shaking palsy' in everyday settings. His acute analysis led to the disease being named after him.[1] This chapter outlines some of the main symptoms of Parkinson's, as well as highlighting issues of treatment and support. In keeping with the objective of the book to foreground the experiences of people with Parkinson's through the voices of people living with the condition, it details the effects these symptoms have on individuals. In doing so, it expands descriptions of symptoms into what lived experiences of those symptoms are like for those with Parkinson's. Most of the voices recorded in this chapter belong to the Parkinson's dancers who participate in English National Ballet's programme in London and Oxford.

Scientists are still studying the pathology that leads to Parkinson's, a common chronic and degenerative condition. The causes of the disease are unknown. There are several theories as to the origin of Parkinson's. Scientists have examined both potential genetic and environmental causes. Some of the ideas being investigated focus on bacteria in the gut and agricultural pesticides. Other studies concentrate on changes happening in the brain. One theory centres on the clumping of alpha-synuclein protein and a depletion of nerve cells in the substantia nigra, a part of the brain within the basal ganglia. As a result, the body gradually loses the chemical dopamine. Dopamine is a neurotransmitter that has several functions and what is clear so far is that post-mortem, brains of those who had Parkinson's show depletion of dopamine. One of its functions is the control of voluntary movement. As dopamine lessens, movement slows down. It becomes difficult to initiate and, conversely, difficult to stop. It is no surprise that Parkinson's is often termed a movement disorder. It

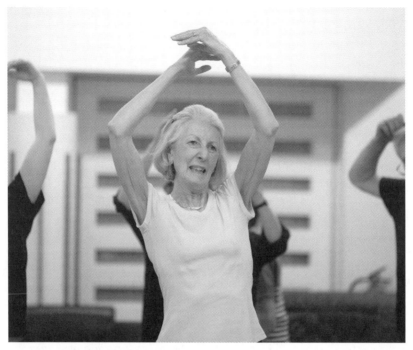

**Figure 1:** English National Ballet Dance for Parkinson's London, photography by Rachel Cherry.

is characterized by the cardinal (or primary) symptoms of a resting tremor, slowness of movement and rigidity of muscles. To be classified as having Parkinson's a person must have at least two of these cardinal symptoms. They are likely to have several other non-motor symptoms too (those not associated with movement).

## Tremor

The primary physical manifestation that people associate with the condition is tremor, although only 70 per cent of people with Parkinson's develop one. As a visible symbol of a lack of control and that something is wrong with the body, tremor can become a source of anxiety. Commonly first found in a hand or foot, the Parkinsonian tremor manifests itself as a small, steady 'pill-rolling' action (Schapira 2008: 17). Characterized as a resting tremor, it is more noticeable when the hand or foot is at rest, than when carrying out an action. It may be more noticeable when the person is stressed or anxious. The tremor may progress to become more violent and intrusive, interfering in people's ability to carry out fine motor tasks, such as fastening a button, writing or holding an object. Pat K (2010) noted that it interfered with her concentration. Roy K (2010) confessed to keeping his hand in his pocket so as to disguise the fact that he had a tremor. The worry about how children might perceive her tremor as frightening, and not knowing how to explain it to them, stopped Josephine DG (2013) helping children read at school. Josephine DG and Roy K's behaviour is not unusual, particularly for people who are newly diagnosed. Anthropologist Samantha Solimeo (2009) notes that tremor often is seen as socially embarrassing by those who develop it, and many place a self-imposed curb on particular social practices. Solimeo describes that some people with Parkinson's decide not to participate in social customs, such as shaking hands, in order to disguise tremor, but then risk being labelled as unfriendly. She highlights one woman who stopped paying for goods with small change as it was too embarrassing getting money out of her purse.

One consequence of dealing with shaking, with trying to concentrate to accomplish tasks or keep on balance, is that it is very tiring, particularly as some medication also encourages somnolence. Josephine DG (2013) wrote in her diary: 'I have been trying to write this all week but half way through each day I flag, fatigued, it's like living a half-life'. Many of Sue C's diary entries begin like this one: 'FATIGUE – dreadful dragging pain in my back, sagging deportment, and completely empty head' (Sue C 2013). Fatigue affects many people with Parkinson's, but it is under-acknowledged (Schulman et al. 2002; EPDA 2014). Palfreman (2015) notes that because of the traditional conception of Parkinson's as a dopamine-deficient movement disorder, clinicians are not so conversant with the non-motor symptoms, particularly as some are challenges for older people in general. In Olsson, Stafström and Söderberg's phenomenological study of fatigue in women with Parkinson's (2013), 42 per cent characterize it as one of the worst symptoms they had developed. The women in this study came to see their body as an unpredictable burden and felt a sense of inertia, unable to function socially as well as before. As Parkinson's fluctuates in intensity, fatigue does also, often appearing without warning.

## Bradykinesia

Movement slowness is technically termed 'bradykinesia' and is another cardinal symptom. Bradykinesia looks like a hesitation within an action, not so much a pause as a lingering over one movement. It is a fragile hesitation, lacking in physical power, and the action may never reach its full conclusion. Josephine DG (2013) writes in her diary: 'I'm slow at everything, bathing, dressing, cooking, thinking. Coffee is cold before I've finished a cup'. Specific manifestations of bradykinesia beyond general slowness are, for example, constipation and facial masking. Constipation is common as digestion slows down, but the urge to empty one's bladder is often heightened. Facial muscles do not work as well, leading to a characteristic mask-like appearance, where expressions of emotions are not readily communicated. Gary, writing to the European Parkinson's Disease Association (EPDA), explains that he does 'not smile easily, my face is stiff and without expression. This can cause misunderstanding when my grandchildren show me their latest book or picture; they cannot see that I am smiling inside' (cited in EPDA 2011: 9).

## Muscular rigidity

Muscular rigidity is the third cardinal symptom. It may manifest itself in cramps and pain. Carroll F (2013) describes the cramps in her right arm and that she has difficulty opening bottles because of them: 'I tried to open a bottle of bleach today and couldn't. It's so frustrating. Even if I want to do the housework I can't'. An associated condition, dystonia, where muscles contract involuntarily, may also present in people with Parkinson's. Jane D'A (2010) describes the feeling of dystonia as 'stiff and starchy'. On another occasion she mentions that 'I'm slow and stiff and my toes feel as if they're curling underneath. I'm not feeling in control' (Jane D'A 2011).

Often stiffness and slowness combine to frustrating ends. The combination of rigidity and bradykinesia leads to a smaller range of movement, which affects both whole body and functional movement. For example, a person with Parkinson's may find it difficult to accomplish fine motor tasks. Paul Q (2012) confesses that his 'hands are not as nimble. I have trouble doing up buttons. It's frustrating. Shoe laces too'. Daily tasks and some physical tasks that were integral to working or pleasure are particularly affected. Some people mention difficulty in washing hair. John H (2012), who had been a successful graphic designer, cannot draw any more. Sue C (2013) explains she gave up playing the organ at her local church because she became 'too disconnected (uncoordinated is the word I'm looking for) between my brain and fingers'. She articulates clearly that even though she knows what she wants to do, her body does not carry out her wishes. For others, muscles that influence swallowing with increased rigidity cause drooling and difficulty in eating, with the added danger of choking.

## Instability

Stiffness and slowness combine to create situations where not only might a person be challenged in completing everyday tasks, but more dangerously where a person is at risk of losing balance. Falling over is a consequence of gait dysfunction and postural instability as Parkinson's progresses. Often a leg will drag, steps become uneven, heels cease to dig into the floor and toes inadequately clear the floor, transforming the walk into a shuffle. Hips, knees and ankles may not bend and flex easily, and the pelvis ceases to be the main driver for leading the body forward. Instead, the chin may lead as the spine starts to curve either forwards or sideways, the chest sinking inward as the neck extends outward. The arms, so important in the rhythmic propulsion and stability of movement, cease to swing: first one, then both as time goes by. The arms are held close to the body, elbows half bent close to the waist as hands stick out forwards. The solidity of the arms is accompanied by stiffness in the torso. A typical walk involves not only the swing of the arms, but also the twisting of the trunk in the opposite direction to the rotation of the pelvis. As muscles become more rigid and arms stop swinging, so the torso stops twisting. Contralateral movement stops and fluid movement becomes harder to accomplish. The eyes often stare ahead, with the head fixed in one position as the person walks, not looking around to be aware of where he or she is going, or to contribute to the delicate art of keeping on balance whilst shifting the weight from one leg to the other. Sometimes festination will develop, as described by Parkinson: uneven steps become quicker, closer together, accelerating until the upper body propels itself forward away from the increasingly smaller yet quicker footsteps until the person is at risk of falling over.

Unexpectedly, their atypical walk does not seem to be so much of a focus when people talk about their symptoms. After all, as Margaret P (2013) commented, 'this is natural to us to walk in this way'. More traumatic is the risk of falling over. Many people express how vulnerable they feel when they realize that their sense of balance has eroded. Charlotte J (2013) expressed it like this: 'I miss balance. Without balance it is terrible, I live in constant fear of falling, I really do. I am terrified of falling. I have dreams about falling. I fall quite often'. Paul M describes a particular situation on the London Underground (known as 'the tube') where losing balance becomes more likely:

> One of the things with Parkinson's is I have become much more aware of gravity. Gravity is quite the enemy really [...]. You've got to get yourself upright and not trip, because that seems to be one of the main things of people with Parkinson's, falling over [...]. Especially the tube, getting off the tube in crowds is quite complex. Once you start noticing people walking in a straight line that goes right through you, they're not going to go around you, you have to slow down and start negotiating space. It can be very disorientating.
>
> (Paul M 2013)

A person's relationship to space changes with the onset of Parkinson's and balance is affected by this. John H describes his specific problem:

> If you're doing something, you've got physical restrictions – buttons, cuffs etc. – it interrupts everything. You have to have focus and so you are oblivious to the things around you. If you focus too much you fall over. I'm a champion of falling over. I've dislocated three fingers. If there are so many surroundings it confuses you. I was staying with my mum in her flat. In the hall there are five doors. It confuses me. I've fallen over there although I didn't tell. She's 99 and she worries about me.
>
> (John H 2012)

## 'Illusions of scale' and disorientation

The disorientation that Paul M feels negotiating crowded spaces and that John H feels when faced with a hallway with five doors manifests itself physically in loss of balance and often in an inability to move. The complex pathways that a typical person would invent to track space through a crowded room, or the quick decisions to dodge sideways, or the ability to take in multiple doorways all at once are not always available to a person with Parkinson's. His or her ability to navigate the world of textures and fluctuating 3D negative and positive spaces can be partial, particularly if his or her eyesight also is deteriorating.

This embodied confusion runs parallel to the shrinking of a person's personal space, or kinesphere. Arms may stick to a person's side as posture droops, steps may become smaller, eye focus may narrow and limbs may fail to stretch out to their extremities. Voices may diminish in strength. Sacks describes this diminishing of space and disorientation, as seen in John H's story, as a case of space-time judgements 'being pushed out of shape' (Sacks [1973] 1990: 344). From time to time perception of space contracts, warps and twists for someone with Parkinson's, causing what Sacks calls 'illusions of scale' (Sacks [1973] 1990: 340) that result in disorientation, loss of balance and gait disturbances. Movement, the occupation of space through time, is distracted by a disjuncture between perception and actual physical motion, as well as the dual, but contradictory, problems of starting and stopping. The brain's confusion translates directly into how people move.

Situations where improvisation is needed and quick thinking and action are necessary require much processing from the brain and a reliance on the body to move and adapt immediately. In these situations, automatic movement, which is achieved without conscious thought, is extremely useful. The basal ganglia, affected in Parkinson's, are tasked with the role of creating automatic movement. These areas of the brain also allow multitasking to happen. Jon Palfreman, a science journalist and a person with Parkinson's, explains the problem:

Having Parkinson's feels a bit like going on vacation in another country and having to drive on the 'wrong' side of the road. Driving is one of those activities that we outsource, in large part, to the basal ganglia [...]. To compensate, the American motorist [driving in Britain] must invoke the conscious, deliberate, mindful, and goal-directed part of his brain – the cortex – to override the basal ganglia. The driving will be difficult, partly because the conscious brain is now doing all the work, but mainly because it's having to compensate for the basal ganglia's signals that are inappropriate for the situation at hand.

(Palfreman 2015: 61)

If the signals are incomplete, misfiring and confused, the body will not respond quickly or effectively to a complicated, moving obstacle course, such as the London Underground at rush hour, or to choosing one of five similar looking doors in a hallway.

One of the most dramatic symptoms allied to festination, disorientation and attempts to multitask is called 'freezing'. A person suddenly feels they cannot move even if they want to. Sacks' patient, Frances D, explained: 'I don't just come to a halt. I am still going, but I *have run out of space to move in*' (cited in Sacks [1973] 1990: 339, original emphasis). Jane D'A (2010) finds it happening to her when going through doorways, from one surface to another: 'All of a sudden you stop and cannot under any circumstances move. It's like a tonne weight on your foot. I'm stuck'. While Frances D links freezing to space contracting, Jane D'A notes the somatic response and the way that texture – moving from one surface to another – may trigger a misjudgement of space. For Pat C, her tendency to freeze has social implications. It is embarrassing: 'If I'm frozen I can't get going and I feel mortified' (Pat C 2012). Charlotte J explains:

> My walking isn't good. I have a very traditional Parkinson's problem, which is walking a few steps and then freezing. I've frozen in the middle of the road. I was crossing in the middle of the road, and the lorry came along and did that to me [makes a gesture to move along], then he flashed his lights at me, then he did this again [does gesture again], then he started swearing at me, then another car came from the other direction, and starting saying this [makes the waving gesture again]. And I was just frozen, I couldn't do anything. It was terrible.
>
> (Charlotte J 2013)

Other people living with Parkinson's echo the embarrassment felt by many of those who freeze. The general public often do not understand particular behaviour symptomatic of Parkinson's and misinterpretation can cause discomfort or humiliation. Renée A has Parkinson's and writes poetry when she cannot sleep at night. She told me about one poem 'Besoffen?' ('Drunk?') which describes an incident she experienced that is typical of many people with Parkinson's, who experience gait dysfunction:

> I called this one 'Drunk' because of people thinking often that I am drunk! That's because of the way I walk in my bad moments as someone with Parkinson's. They may think whatever they want, but I was shocked when people I don't know and who don't know me asked me on the street why I am drinking so much. The fact is that I was never drunk in my whole life! That's unbelievable! Must I explain the way I am walking? A few weeks ago a man of my age, I was shopping […] and he past me and looked at me from top to toe, you know what I mean, and then he observed me for a while and he was gone. But after a few minutes someone behind me whispered in my ear: 'Hey Beauty, why do you drink so much? That's not good for you!' And then he walked away! Can you imagine that?
>
> (Renée A 2014)

Hanna, featured in an EPDA support booklet, suggests a solution for people misinterpreting the cause of imbalanced movement and slurred words: 'To wear a badge that says "I am not drunk, I have Parkinson's" would be a good idea' (cited in EPDA 2011: 28). As Hanna and Renée A's experience suggests, the symptoms of Parkinson's create situations that may be embarrassing or degrading, or where others, ignorant of their condition, may make moral judgements. Experiences may also be funny, mundane or life-enhancing, but it is clear from the stories people tell that Parkinson's attracts more than its fair share of negative experiences.

## Cognitive challenges and mental health

Some aspects of Parkinson's are not always immediately visible. The link between cognitive slowness or impairment and Parkinson's is one that Parkinson himself failed to categorize. As movement slows, so can thought processes, particularly those concerning executive function – planning, decision-making and goal-orientated tasks. Sue C (2013) writes in her diary that one day her brain was 'completely unable to cope with texting and emailing', and she got frustrated. Another time she mentions a 'completely empty head' (Sue C 2013). Many people mention slowness in retrieving words and recalling how to do things. Mary C (2011) explains, 'with Parkinson's the words don't come. They come five minutes later'. A high proportion of people with mild-cognitive impairment progress to Parkinsonian dementia (Litvan et al. 2011), which many fear. Christine B acknowledges that she worries about the future. She confesses to be 'undergoing memory assessments and it's a bit traumatic. If anything is diagnosed I hope that I can find a way of dealing with it' (Christine B 2012). Josephine DG writes her diary at night when she cannot sleep and poetically describes actions she takes to remember things:

> Sleep is elusive. The nightmares are bad sometimes, dreams are crowded. Thoughts flit, I need to catch them on Post-it notes before they are gone. Then try to arrange them so I know what I have to do [...]. Sometimes I think I can feel my brain cells shrinking, I reach for a word, it has gone beyond reach.
>
> (Josephine DG 2013)

As well as talking about the difficulty of grasping words, Josephine DG also mentions difficulty sleeping, which often is an early symptom in Parkinson's. Night-time is a time of restlessness and even, for some, terror. Many people with Parkinson's do not sleep for long, a few hours at most and often many cannot turn in bed. Dreams and hallucinations may break through to consciousness. Some hallucinations are brought on by medication. Clare N (2010) changed hers after perceiving three big dogs in her bedroom. Yet some bad dreams seem to afflict those with Parkinson's irrespective of medication. Acting out dreams is also common and often a hazard for partners sleeping in the same bed. Josephine DG gives a vivid picture of her dreams:

> I have developed a new type of nightmare, and now have three. The first is the straightforward, nasty terrifying nightmare, the second, the screaming nightmare. Anybody within hearing distance wakes me up from one of these [...]. Now I've developed the sleepwalking nightmare. The night before last I woke to find myself standing by the side of the wardrobe in my bedroom, trying to open it as though it was a very stiff door, in order to escape from a monster in the garage of a house I thought I still lived in.
>
> (Josephine DG 2013)

Far from being just a movement disorder, Parkinson's reaches into the dark corners of the mind, retrieving fears that usually remain buried.

It is perhaps no surprise that one common, often debilitating, effect of Parkinson's is the onset of depression. Around 40 per cent of people with Parkinson's develop depression (Cummings 1992). Ray P (2012b) talked about his depression in these terms: 'I used to lie in bed and cry. Why is this happening? I couldn't make sense of it. It was like I was taken over by an alien force'. Schulman et al. (2002) note that many doctors under-diagnose non-motor symptoms, such as depression, anxiety, fatigue and sleep disorders, and thus overlook the consequential reduction in their patients functioning well.

## Treatment and support

One consequence of the complexity of the disease, which has so many diverse symptoms (van der Marck et al. 2009), is that doctors often struggle to treat patients effectively (Solimeo 2009). Not everyone develops all symptoms, and many people acquire new ones during the course of their lifetime. Degeneration is more aggressive in some than in others. Individuals respond in different ways to both symptoms and medication, so much so that there is a suggestion that there may be more than one disease that we are dealing with. Even in one person, Parkinson's does not get *steadily* worse but is unpredictable in the strength and pace of its trajectory. Carroll F (2012a) calls it 'quixotic'. People find they have good hours and bad hours; good days and bad days; good months and bad months. Many think that extremes of weather affect symptoms and emotional stress is particularly influential in exacerbating them.

In order to treat Parkinsonian symptoms there are a number of different medicines, but Levodopa, or L-dopa, is the primary form of medication. First administered experimentally in 1960s, patients now usually take it in conjunction with other drugs.[2] People with Parkinson's often remark on Levodopa's effectiveness to lessen bradykinesia in particular. But the medication loses its effectiveness after several years, and with this lessening comes the experience of 'on' and 'off' states. When in an 'on' state, a person with Parkinson's can function fairly well – the medication is working. When in an 'off' state, Parkinsonian symptoms may dominate functionality – the medication is not working. Writing about his own Parkinsonian condition, Cecil Todes describes the 'on' period as a time when 'one is tricked into feeling normal and even athletic and that it will last' (1990: 58). He describes the 'off' period as 'depressing and a reminder of failure' (1990: 58) and 'ultimately soul-destroying' (1990: 99).

It is challenging to find the optimal dose and brand of medication that suits the particular person in order to increase its effectiveness and lessen side effects. There are some common side effects from different medication, some of which are challenging to deal with. For example, as pointed out above, hallucinations can be one; impulsive and compulsive behaviours are others (often for activities, such as gambling and sex, which may become high risk through compulsive use). Over-medication of Levodopa may lead to involuntary movement called dyskinesia. Instead of a slow moving stiffness, people with dyskinesia may move with a destabilizing wildness, heads, torsos and arms each completing their own elliptical trajectories. Alternatively, dyskinesia may present itself, for example, at first in the shoulders, hands and fingers: twitching fingers pulling into the body, a shoulder pulling up towards the neck. Alan F has dyskinesia for four to five hours during the day and it gets worse for him at night. He says: 'I notice I can get up and I can buck like a scarecrow in a windstorm. It's very anxiety provoking walking down the street [...] I have noticed how awkward I felt' (Alan F 2013). Many people lose weight with the continuous movement, but many prefer to be dyskinetic than stuck without much movement at all.

## Care: Burdens and barriers

Beyond the challenge of treating people with Parkinson's effectively lies the problem of access to medical help and information. For the *Move for Change* report, people living with Parkinson's in 35 European countries were asked questions on standards of care between 2010 and 2013. The report found that 44 per cent of patients never see a Parkinson's specialist and only 18 per cent see a specialist Parkinson's nurse regularly (EPDA 2014). Other paramedical services, such as those offered by speech therapists, social workers and dieticians, were 'largely unavailable' (EPDA 2014). These results are backed up by research carried out by Nijkrake and colleagues (2010) in the Netherlands, who in response set up ParkinsonsNet, a visible and accessible network of health care and allied therapy specialists for people living with Parkinson's across the country. The situation detailed by the EPDA and Nijkrake and colleagues goes hand in hand with the lack of information given to patients on diagnosis. The *Move to Change* report noted that on diagnosis, less than 3 per cent of respondents received information about Parkinson's support organizations (EPDA 2014).

Chronic disease can be a large financial burden on health and welfare systems, and health economic policies may bring challenges. As a result, people with Parkinson's can find that the level of support they need is not always in place. In countries, such as the United States, where health insurance is expensive, many people on fixed incomes struggle with the rising cost of medication and living with the condition (Solimeo 2009). In the United Kingdom, specialist Parkinson's nurses are highly valued by people living with Parkinson's, but provision can be inconsistent, with some local health budgets leaning towards providing generalist health care professionals, rather than specialists. Family members often fall into the role of caregivers, finding their job all consuming, with hardly any respite or recompense (Ephgrave 2010).

The estimated economic cost of the disease in Europe alone is €13.9 billion (EPDA 2014). Each country shows slightly different costs depending on the budgets set by individual governments, but the economic burden is high. For example, in a cost of living report (Gumber et al. 2017), people with Parkinson's in England pay an extra £17,094 per year due to higher health costs. These include prescriptions, travel to see medical professionals and mobility aids. There are also higher social care costs, which include home alterations, help with cleaning and shopping and equipment to stay independent, as well as loss of income as work stops or reduces, and a lower quality of life. At the beginning of the twenty-first century, approximately one in 500 have Parkinson's (Parkinson's UK 2014), but the number of people developing the condition is set to double by 2030 (EPDA 2014). As a result, the economic cost of the disease will escalate.

The personal cost of developing Parkinson's can be high too. Leonora (2011) comments that 'it wears you out and breaks you down'. Despite this, some people with Parkinson's try to live a fulfilling life in spite of, or alongside, having Parkinson's. In a letter to the EPDA, Szentes Béla says: 'To help me fight this battle I am involved with various activities, have a good social life and regular work. I read, write, listen to and play music, walk, hike and in summer time I garden' (cited in EPDA 2011: 15). David Sangster, a school teacher from Bolton, United Kingdom, diagnosed at the age of 29, decided to advocate for young people who develop Parkinson's. In 2015, despite working and having a young family, he set up the Young Parkinson's Network to harness positivity, engagement and support. He is passionate about spreading the idea that people with Parkinson's can have positive, fulfilling lives. Sacks notes, '[t]he central problem in all Parkinsonian disorders is *passivity* – passivity and pulsivity, i.e. inertia – as the central cure for them all is *activity* (of the right kind)' ([1973] 1990: 345). The *Move for Change* report highlighted the importance of 'patient-centred care' (EPDA 2014: 40) in which people with Parkinson's play an active role in their own management of their condition, alongside their physician and allied health professionals. The report cited several studies suggesting that patients who take ownership over managing the disease demonstrate 'better clinical outcomes, improved treatment adherence, greater quality of life and lower healthcare costs' (EPDA 2014: 40). For some people with Parkinson's, this does not just mean making a joint decision about medication with their physician, it also means deciding which activities might be interesting and beneficial for them to do in order to help with well-being and quality of life. Van der Marck et al. (2009) argue that care for people with Parkinson's has to be multidisciplinary, and addressed in different ways, not just through pharmacological treatments as these are insufficient to the task of holistic care. Van der Marck et al. (2009) suggest that dancing might be an effective strategy to help with daily functioning, one means of complementing standard medical treatments. As Chapter 2 shows, dancing has become an activity embedded in the lives of many people who are living with Parkinson's.

## Notes

1  Throughout the book, I use the term 'Parkinson's' rather than 'Parkinson's disease' or 'PD'. Although the latter two terms are in common use in North America, particularly in research journals, 'Parkinson's' is the preferred term amongst the Parkinson's community in the United Kingdom and in other countries. Describing it as a 'condition' (that one lives

with) rather than a disease is favoured too. In addition, the term 'PD' is used by the UK medical community to mean 'personality disorder' not 'Parkinson's disease'. Since much of the primary research featured here focuses on the experiences of UK-based individuals with Parkinson's, I will use their preferred term throughout.

2   Some patients try other interventions, such as deep brain stimulation. DBS, as it is known as, requires surgery to place an electrode, or electrodes, in the brain in order to lessen tremor. Not all patients are deemed suitable for this surgical intervention.

# Chapter 2

The phenomenon of dance for Parkinson's

D ance for Parkinson's is a global phenomenon, growing exponentially since the early 2000s. Classes, programmes and workshops are seen in many countries over several continents. This chapter details several successful approaches to provision and maps out some of the artistic networks that have supported the development of dance for Parkinson's. The chapter argues that, alongside the recognition that dancing may be of benefit to people living with Parkinson's, these networks and approaches have facilitated a rippling out of provision worldwide.

The chapter situates the phenomenon within the broader community dance movement and specifically within arts in community health provision. It argues that the values and approaches used within community dance and arts in community health are echoed within much dance for Parkinson's practice. These values and approaches (with much of the scholarship and development of practice emanating from the United Kingdom) are important to highlight because they create the distinguishing characteristics of dance for Parkinson's, as well as a tradition of practice that reaches back further than the first dance for Parkinson's sessions. They are discussed below, alongside descriptions of the major approaches to facilitation and teaching and some of the networks of support and development. Specific classes and programmes are used to illustrate the characteristics of dance for Parkinson's and how approaches to facilitation work in practice.

Drawn from interviews with teaching artists and from my attendance at dance for Parkinson's classes and events from 2010 onwards, the account reflects my own engagement, not just as a researcher, but also increasingly as an actor in events. In 2014 I became chair of the initial steering group of the Dance for Parkinson's Network UK (now known as the Dance for Parkinson's Partnership UK) and so I have taken part in decisions on the strategic course of dance for Parkinson's in the United Kingdom. In addition, I have been called upon as a researcher with an overview of practice internationally to help develop dance provision and facilitation in this area and to speak on behalf of the dance for Parkinson's community. The line between objective researcher and involved player is therefore blurred. It is perhaps not surprising that researchers in a fledgling specialist practice are more involved in outcomes than in more established situations.[1] The following account focuses on the voices of dance teaching artists, rather than my own, but necessarily it is a narrative inflected by my own experience.

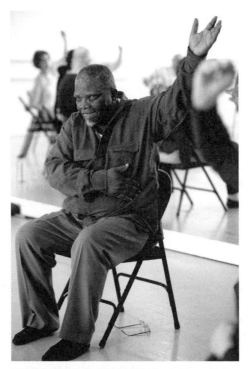

**Figure 2:** Dance for PD at Mark Morris Dance Group, photography by Rosalie O'Connor.

## A note on barriers to dancing

Before discussing the global dance for Parkinson's movement and describing the provision and teaching available, it is important to point out that there are barriers to dancing in general for older people and for people living with Parkinson's. It is important to note because in advocating for dance for Parkinson's it is easy for the problems to go unacknowledged. Additionally, it is worth highlighting the issues in order to understand that not being able to dance is connected to social assumptions and lack of access, rather than an innate lack of skill or ability. Access may be problematic if there is no local dance class. It is often hard for people with Parkinson's to travel a long way as this is tiring and expensive. Moreover, apathy, as well as other symptoms that may flair up, makes it even more difficult to get out of the house to dance. Sometimes there are general dance classes, but not with a teacher that is sympathetic to the needs of someone with Parkinson's. Sometimes the building is not accessible for those coming in a wheelchair or with a walking frame or stick. Other barriers include the assumptions people may hold about who dances. Dance is seen as a young person's activity and an activity for those who are fit, co-ordinated, flexible and strong. That assumption means that those who are older and/or who are less agile are not so likely to choose to dance.

For those who are young but with Parkinson's, they do not necessarily want to be reminded they have an 'old person's disease' and dance with more mature people with Parkinson's; for those who are newly diagnosed, they do not necessarily want to be reminded of their future and dance in the company of those with more progressed Parkinson's. Culturally, there may be taboos on dancing or on dancing with those of another gender.

## Community and participatory dance provision

The dance for Parkinson's initiative owes much to the influence of the community dance movement. Community dance aims to engage communities and individuals in dancing, which is often, but certainly not exclusively, led by professional dance teaching artists. The community dance movement embraces the idea that anyone may dance, irrespective of training, age, gender, ability, social circumstance or cultural background, and that a person's way of dancing is to be respected, whatever their ability or whatever genre of dance they undertake. Ken Bartlett, an influential British community dance commentator, argues that the community dance movement has developed a set of values that 'include a belief that everybody can dance with intention and purpose; that we build on what people bring to the engagement [...]. We build on what people *can* do, rather than what they can't achieve' (Bartlett 2008: 40, original emphasis). According to this view, community dance facilitation is a process that values and respects each individual and his or her abilities through the medium of artistic practice. The individual's way of moving is valued above a pedantic adherence to a particular dance technique, which may impose movement constraints on them. Different dance forms have specific ways of moving and specific technical rules about how to move. These rules often set the standard by which to measure 'good' or 'bad' dancing in any form. A teaching artist may want to teach these rules in a way that asks the dancer to fit into the aesthetic, even if the rules are challenging, rather than seeing what the dancer might bring to the tradition in which they are working. Bartlett's notion of 'building on' demonstrates how community dance proponents start from what the individual brings to the class, not necessarily from what the teaching artist thinks is appropriate before meeting their participants.

In this way, community dance is a person-centred practice that aims to be inclusive in its outlook and practices. Sue Akroyd, a community dance commentator, argues that this approach develops 'relationships based on common ground, mutual respect, responsibility and trust' (1996:17). Akroyd describes this way of working as 'the social imperative' within people-centred dance. This stance lends itself well to teaching those who might not necessarily want to, or be able to, learn how to dance within a mainstream setting, where the teacher might be more didactic and less willing to accommodate individual concerns, ideas and abilities. Indeed, dance scholar Jill Green argues that 'community dance has often been linked to disenfranchised populations such as the elderly [...] those with special needs and physical disabilities, those with health needs and "at risk" children' (2000: 54). Anthropologist Kate Crehan notes a similar tendency within community practice in visual arts:

> Within the visual arts, community art encompassed a general sense of an art that was not gallery art, that was collective rather than individual, and that addressed itself to those living in 'areas of deprivation' not normally reached by the established arts.
>
> (Crehan 2011: 81)

Although community dance has more of a distinct emphasis on the participant as an individual within the collective, Crehan's description fits well. Community teaching artists, including those from dance, have been ignited by the idea that art can be democratized, particularly to include those who might otherwise not have access to artistic experiences. Dance for Parkinson's initiatives arguably fit into a democratized view of dance, where those who initially may feel they are not able to dance because of increasing disability, or who would feel out of place in a mainstream dance class, are given the opportunity to dance. For example, Alan F remarks that he would not go to a club to dance and 'wouldn't be able to go to ballroom as I'm too self-conscious' and yet being given the chance to express himself 'is very important' (in discussion group 2014b).

The characteristics of community dance and community arts in general are more nuanced and less uniform than the picture above gives. There are two contrasting interpretations of the democratization of art and dance provision. The debate focuses on two differing concepts of what the expression 'democracy' might mean, in terms of engaging with communities through art. In his polemical text, Owen Kelly, a community arts practitioner and activist, cites two distinct uses of the word in connection to community arts practices: the 'democratization of culture' and 'cultural democracy' (1984: 100). In the democratization of culture, the arts as made by professional artists are brought as a ready-made package to the people. A dance company performing an extract from a dance work, then teaching a class and giving insights into the work at a local school would be one example. The democratization of culture entails that the arts, as made by professional artists, are brought to audiences and participants in a way that enables them to experience them and to be informed about them. Peter Brinson's Ballet for All company that toured Britain in the 1960s with 'ballet plays' of words, music and dance to increase appreciation of ballet works by the general public, is one such early initiative in dance education (Brinson and Crisp 1970). In contrast, cultural democracy gives communities the tools to create their own artistic means of expression. Kelly describes cultural democracy as revolving 'around equality of access to the means of cultural production and distribution' (1984: 101). Community arts, which are founded in cultural democracy, encourage the participants to take ownership of what is being made, how it is executed and how it is displayed. His approach echoes that of Sherry R. Arnstein (1969), who formulated a 'ladder' of participation and agency as conceived by organizations for the active citizen. From manipulation and therapy to informing and consultation, through to placation and partnership, and then to delegated power and citizen control, the ladder moves towards the handover of power to the citizen.

Claire Bishop (2012) points out that the argument from the 1980s onwards swung in favour of those who wanted to democratize culture, away from those more radical artists who wanted a culture of democracy. In the 1980s the political climate in several first-world countries, including Britain, veered towards promoting a neo-liberal market economy. The consequence for performing arts organizations in the United Kingdom was that they were encouraged to commodify art that was produced, in other words, to create outputs that had economic value. Commodification included engagement with people who wanted to participate in creating art. One consequence has been to frame participation in the arts, as offered by organizations, as a means to an end, often where participants are seen as beneficiaries (Jancovich 2015), or even customers, whether it be for marketing a company's performance programme, for contributing to the regeneration of a deprived area, or to aiding a person's physical health.[2] Bringing culture to the people (democratization of culture) can comfortably fit into a vision where art is created as monetary gain, or for other instrumental value. It is arguably more difficult to fit into this vision when the demand for culture is created by grassroots action, where participants are not commodities, but agents for participatory action, as in a culture of democracy.

The reality for most organizations, particularly those who are either funded publicly, or who are funded through private funding with a specific societal remit, is that in order to survive with the help of these grants, they usually have to make an explicit claim that they are doing socially relevant work.[3] Moreover, with projects that are for people with specific health conditions, there is great temptation to claim that because they are for people with a health condition, the project is automatically beneficial and socially relevant. There is tension between needing to advocate for the arts as being important and beneficial in general and admitting that the specificities of individual arts projects may or may not be high quality, or involve participatory processes that create inclusion or empowerment. Arts policy scholar Jonathan Price points out that,

> there is little incentive to publicly challenge the received wisdom of participation's supposed virtues within a sector for which participatory work is a key part of the economy and which invests in promoting its benefits.
>
> (Price 2015: 20)

The advocacy and belief in the power of the arts has sustained and covered divergent practices that Kelly in particular was so keen to separate.

As well as attracting an instrumental approach to engagement, the democratization of culture can also attract a specific style of pedagogy. Dance, as seen within the teaching traditions of many classical, modern, contemporary and popular forms, has a history of education that sits within what educationalist Paulo Freire calls the 'banking model' (1993: 53). In Freire's colourful description, the banking model is characterized as a transmission of knowledge from master to pupil. Much mainstream participation in dance, either at a professional or community level, is often experienced as a process of banking. The transference of knowledge from master to pupil establishes a hierarchy of power, as seen within some of Arnstein's descriptions of participation and similarly in Jo Butterworth's dance teaching and leading grid (2009). So, for example, although there has been a long-established tradition of community dance in the United Kingdom, much mainstream work has imitated the longstanding traditions where unequal power structures have been entrenched in how many people learn to dance. Although also critiqued within the British community dance sector, the democratization of culture is sometimes far from espousing a flattened hierarchy or equality of engagement.

Community dance commentators have laid out their version of Kelly's notions of democratizing the arts. Chris Thomson (1994) proposes three types of community dance practice: 'alternative', 'ameliorative' and 'radical'. The 'alternative' emphasizes a holistic approach incorporating the execution of the physical with therapy for the mind and the practice links to other complementary and therapeutic services. The 'radical', in contrast, emphasizes empowerment for participants to overcome discrimination or oppression. It is based around ideas of community action, and the activity often is associated with social welfare provision. Thus, radical community dance helps participants challenge the institutional order where it has failed them in some way. The 'ameliorative' promotes the participant's sense of well-being, of having fun, and offers a wide range of dance activity. It is often associated with recreation and leisure and, as a result, is 'well-integrated into [the] economic and institutional order' (Thomson 1994: 25).

Freire's banking model often could be applied to ameliorative or indeed alternative notions of community dance, although not always. Kelly's notion of democratization of culture is invoked in this tradition, where dance is taught *to* people. Many dance commentators would substitute the word 'community' for 'participatory' in this context to underscore the focus on participating versus that of community building, where change or a shift of perspective might happen *through* dance, or where dance is used *by* people to create something together.[4] Youth dance expert Linda Jasper clearly distinguishes between community building and mainstream participatory dance. She argues that there are 'distinctive working principles that seem directly to address the concept of dance as a medium for community development, and in particular the individual within the community' (Jasper 1995: 187). The majority of community dance, however, may be termed ameliorative. Dance for Parkinson's initiatives may fit into radical, ameliorative or alternative categories of practice and develop along the lines of Freire's banking model, or as part of a community's cultural democracy. Teaching styles likewise may suit a variety of points along Butterworth or Arnstein's spectrum of power in leadership.

## Arts in community health

Nestled within the practices of community arts is a strand that is often referred to as 'arts in community health' where the arts exist alongside, within and through community health practices and institutions. In his authoritative account, Mike White (2009), medical humanities scholar and community arts practitioner, considers 'community health' as a broad term to define not just the physical, mental and emotional health of individuals living in a locality, but the social health of those communities as well. White defines this area of arts practice as facilitating 'the experience of well-being among people who are in poor health, or at risk of it, by means of communal involvement in creative activities' (2009: 1). As a strand of community arts activity, arts in community health more often than not puts its focus on the art, rather than specifically on improving health or combatting illness, which are usually associated with arts therapy (Macnaughton et al. 2005).[5] Arts in community health practitioners argue that focusing on the art can help develop health within communities and for individuals. White notes, '[t]hrough sustained programmes of participatory arts, shared creativity can make committed expressions of public health, simultaneously identifying and addressing the local and specific health needs in a community' (2009: 4). He argues that this happens within community art-making through the encouragement of social interaction and through supporting the growth of positive expressions of identity throughout life.

> The consolation of art has often been its ability to support this kind of adaptation at the very edge of human experience. Art can be a potent medium for expressing health – and indeed ill health and distress – and an emphasis on creative messaging is often found at the core of arts in community health.
>
> (White 2009: 4)

He points out that this focus links arts in community health work to social inclusion and aligns it with a social model of health, rather than a medical model (White 2009). Arts in community health does not deal necessarily with ailment and disease, but with bringing people together to produce a positive creative endeavour that may encourage new attitudes towards ailments, self-identity and communal identity. Dance for Parkinson's can be seen as affiliating broadly with White's definition of arts in community health, where the emphasis on artistic, communal practice eclipses focus on disease and illness. It is an emphasis that I advocate for within later chapters in this book.

## A major US initiative: Dance for PD, a lead dance for Parkinson's organization

> We face each other. One group on one side of the studio – the Jets – face the Sharks on the other side. In the corner, the pianist plays the introduction to Bernstein's iconic music of the meeting of the two rival gangs in the musical theatre production *West Side Story*. Each group moves forward in time, starting crouching, gradually raising the body, stepping forward, raising hands to click fingers. Each person looks at someone opposite. Gradually we meet each other in the centre of the studio. The piano crashes three chords and each person punches the air with their own three poses.
>
> (Houston field notes, Dance for PD, Mark Morris Dance Center 2011)

In New York, United States, in 2001, the programme featured above began. It would be a major player in triggering the worldwide dance for Parkinson's movement. In 2017, there were affiliated programmes in more than twenty countries (Dance for PD 2017). The establishment of the programme is a story of collaboration between an internationally acclaimed dance company and a small, local community group. The ensemble-focused contemporary dance company, the Mark Morris Dance Group (MMDG), moved its headquarters to a new building in the Brooklyn area of the city. Already working with schools there, MMDG was committed to sharing its space with the local community (Nichols 2010). An advert in the *New York Times* inviting proposals of collaboration attracted the eye of the enterprising organizer of the newly formed Brooklyn Parkinson Group, Olie Westheimer.

Westheimer was clear in her vision that the Brooklyn Parkinson Group should be founded on non-disease-related activities. With a passion for the arts, and for dance in particular, Westheimer wanted to develop an arts programme that could be enjoyed by people living with Parkinson's (Westheimer 2011). A chance remark from her husband, neurologist Ivan Bodis-Wallner, that people with Parkinson's have to think about how to do actions in order to carry them out, set her thinking. Westheimer knew that in a dance class, a teacher will break down a step, or phrase of movements, into little sections so that it is easier for the pupil to learn and remember. She concluded that to carry out activities, people with Parkinson's have to think like a dancer, breaking movement down in order to do one section at a time and complete the activity. She said that this 'idea was just sitting in my head. Who was going to listen to me? And I had no money' (Westheimer 2010). MMDG's newspaper advert was timely and spurred her on. MMDG embraced Westheimer's idea and not only provided and funded company dancers (John Heginbotham and David Leventhal) to teach the class, a studio to dance in and a pianist (William Wade) to play, but also took on the management and administration of the dance programme, with Leventhal eventually becoming its director. The programme was named Dance for PD ('PD' stands for Parkinson's disease).

Dance for PD takes as its starting point adapted material from the MMDG repertory, as well as elements of ballet and tap dance, and the idea of telling stories through dance. The class consists of a mixture of carefully explained exercises where the movement is broken down and explained before dancing, follow-my-leader exercises where participants follow the teaching artist whilst doing the exercise and participant-led improvisation. It follows a three-tiered structure: first, exercises performed seated on chairs in a circle, then standing exercises holding onto a *barre* or the back of a chair and finally dancing across the floor. The class always finishes in a circle again with an acknowledgement, or 'reverence', to each fellow participant.

Now boasting over 60 members who attend one or two dance sessions a week at Mark Morris Dance Center, Dance for PD also delivers classes for anyone living with Parkinson's across New York, including at the time of writing two in Manhattan, one in the Queens area and two in the Bronx/Riverside areas. The class in the Manhattan West Side takes place at the Juilliard School. As with Mark Morris Dance Center, the Juilliard School offers a place where there are professionally orientated dance activities happening alongside community participation. In the case of Juilliard, young students, training for professional dance careers, and people with Parkinson's, many in their eighth or ninth decade, mix in a building housing purpose-built dance studios and social spaces.

Westheimer's vision of a dance programme that is not about disease but about art, is clearly distilled not only in the focus on MMDG repertory, but also in the deliberate use of venues that hothouse artistic knowledge, understanding and production, such as the Julliard School and Mark Morris Dance Center. Dance for PD is an artistic venture, rather than an initiative that is grounded in the notion of therapy for the sick person. The idea that the class is offered as a therapy to treat Parkinson's is vehemently refuted by Westheimer, Heginbotham and Leventhal. Leventhal recalls: 'Olie [Westheimer] didn't want it as therapy. She tried to shield us from the medical side of things. We didn't want to teach to the symptoms' (Leventhal 2010). Instead, the class is a place where participants 'could leave it [Parkinson's] at the door' (Leventhal 2010). In fact, over the years, the Dance for PD teaching team has accumulated a great deal of knowledge and understanding of how Parkinson's affects their participants, but their approach within the studio remains clearly on dance. Leventhal explains that participants enjoy the artistic focus that Dance for PD offers, which is distinct from the way Parkinson's dominates their everyday lives:

> Participants spend so much time talking and thinking about PD [...] because they all share a similar reality and identity, but they don't want to talk about it [...]. We have a break during class so I might ask Judy how she's doing. 'Well my back really hurts, my balance is bad. But I don't want to talk about that, I'm in a dance class'.
>
> (Leventhal 2010)

Leventhal compares Judy's situation with being on stage, explaining that the experience of dancing is about being in the present moment, not dwelling on what has happened that day, or during the week. As an intangible art form, dance is ideally placed to offer a moment in time, which is all about the present: about imagining and focusing on moving the body in real time.

Emphasizing the notion that dancing aims not to reduce symptoms, but is offered for its own sake, the approach provides scope for the articulation of the aesthetic, 'rather than mechanical, clinical or practical goals' (Dance for PD 2011: 6). For Leventhal, using the MMDG repertory, which enables the creation of stories, is one key to structuring the aesthetic within Dance for PD:

> When you give people a story, the brain and imagination and body are supported by that activity. The imagination creates a road map for the body to walk into. Once you layer a story you feel connected to it in a way, which you don't with abstract movement.
>
> (Leventhal 2010)

Above all, telling stories is fun to do. Much of the MMDG repertory illustrates dance's capacity for joy through storytelling, and as a community arts activity, Dance for PD anchors its practice in joy (Bee 2008).

Dance scholar Joan Acocella (1998) suggests that Morris' aesthetic is partly informed by the celebration of humanness. His group of performers are a collection of people with fairly different body shapes, heights and ages. He encourages them to move with weight and effort, or 'non-effortlessness' (Morris cited in Acocella 1998: 275), which allows the spectator to see the visceral, fleshy vulnerability of people trying to do things. Acocella describes this in relation to Morris' interest in displaying the buttocks:

> To Morris they [the buttocks] seem to represent something modest and tender and unacknowledged, the body's vulnerability. At the same time, what they represent in dance terms is the body's dignity, for they are the motor of action […]. So in both senses the buttocks harbor a fundamental truth, and one that in Morris's eyes is validated by the fact that it requires exposure. For him, truth is always hard to find. Veils have to be dropped.
>
> (Acocella 1998: 270–71)

The exposure of the engines of movement and the emotional vulnerability of being human through this exposure partly create Morris' aesthetic. It is interesting to note this in the light of the company's work with the Brooklyn Parkinson Group, with people who expose their effort in moving in all its human vulnerability. The aesthetic of human effort, vulnerability and joy is perhaps at the heart of the partnership's success. Both organizations and the people involved understand the inflections of the aesthetic because it speaks to those who strive to move: both the professional MMDG dancers and those with Parkinson's.

### Dance for PD's training for dance artists

Dance for PD has attracted much attention for its Brooklyn Parkinson Group programme. The efforts of Westheimer in talking about the dance sessions and conducting research (Westheimer 2008; Westheimer et al. 2015) have been matched by several powerful films (see for example Bee 2008; Iverson 2014a), documentary features and other media coverage that have disseminated information about the venture. Members of the Dance for PD team also have presented their vision and approach to teaching to several World Parkinson Congresses, the largest international gathering of Parkinson's researchers, activists, people living with the condition and medical professionals, which meets biennially to further knowledge and understanding. Leventhal and Westheimer were co-recipients of the Alan Bonander Humanitarian Award in 2013 for their work with people with Parkinson's. It is a successful, high-profile initiative, but it has been its training programme for teaching artists and allied professionals that arguably has generated a worldwide dance for Parkinson's movement. Between 2007 and 2014, over 600 people from seventeen countries attended Dance for PD training programmes (Dance for PD 2014). Delegates take part in a variety of workshops, seminars, experiential laboratories and classes to develop their knowledge and understanding of facilitating dance for people living with Parkinson's. Training is certified and trained teaching artists may use the Dance for PD trademarked logo to advertise their classes.

The training programme has opened up opportunities for dance for Parkinson's classes to be run around the world and using local dance cultures. Kathak dancer Vonita Singh was interested in running both a support group and dance for Parkinson's sessions in her home city of Dubai, United Arab Emirates (Singh 2014). Singh's late father had Parkinson's, and she recognized the importance of movement to people with the condition, but Parkinson's is a hidden disease in Dubai because the stigma attached to the condition is great. Initially, the neuro-spinal hospitals and clinics did not want to help. Singh could find no Parkinson's support groups in Dubai and no activities tailored for people with Parkinson's. She wanted to reach out to people with Parkinson's but did not know how to connect. In 2013 Singh attended the Dance for PD training programme in New York. In talking to others there, she devised a new strategy, finding people with Parkinson's living in Dubai through social media sites, such as Facebook. The training programme also gave Singh the tools to use Kathak, the north Indian classical dance form in which she is trained, within a Dance for PD system of working. Singh recounts, 'I went to New York not sure of what and how. When I came back, I realized I had been given the responsibility to use and carry out the form that I knew' (Singh 2014). In other words, the approach to facilitation in Dance for PD work is more important than the form of dance used. Her support group and dance sessions are still small, but with the continued help and encouragement from the Dance for PD teaching team, she has several plans to enhance the visibility and grow the acceptability of Parkinson's in Dubai and to teach dance classes.

Through the Dance for PD network, Singh was able to visit a programme set up in Pune, India, by Hrishikesh Pawar. Pawar is trained in Kathak as well as in western contemporary dance forms, which he studied in Dresden, Germany. He wanted to work in India with a contemporary dance idiom, but found a lack of interest for this type of dance work. So, Pawar decided to curate a dance film festival in the hope of creating an appetite for contemporary dance. Dance for PD gave him permission to show a film about the Brooklyn Parkinson class. This initial contact with Dance for PD inspired Pawar to establish his own dance group for people with Parkinson's.

Aware of the cultural differences between Pune and New York, he has not attempted to model the Dance for PD approach, but rather to establish a programme that takes into account people's cultural tastes and habits, as well as his own interests as an artist. For example, the dance class uses rhythms and percussive movements found in Kathak. Participants cook and celebrate the long Hindu festivals together, and they write daily reflective passages on their relationship to movement, a practice that Pawar has taken from his own artistic labour. Over eight years, the programme has grown from three participants to over 35 people, some of whom visit Pune for only a few weeks a year. Pawar maintains that the reason the class has grown in popularity (and fame) is that he has encouraged artistic challenge. It is not a therapy class run out of pity. He states, 'we never look at participants and say, "this is so, so bad" [...]. We pull and push the envelope to a high. They can do it. I like to teach that to facilitators. It's the reason it's grown. We've never ever sat down and said, "oh poor you"' (Pawar 2015). Pawar's vision has allowed him to develop artistic practice with those who know movement challenge well.

Dorothy (Dottie) Beaton, Roberta (Bert) Risch and Jane McDonald also know this challenge. Both Risch and McDonald have Parkinson's, and Beaton's mother had it. These three women are examples of how the Dance for PD programme trains not only professional dance artists, but also those with Parkinson's who have a life-long interest in dance. Beaton, Risch and McDonald set up dance classes for people with Parkinson's in Cape Cod, United States. McDonald recalls:

> I had been tap dancing for 18 years. I went to the Doctor's because one night when I came home from tap class, I told my husband something was wrong because I was having difficulty with the steps. I was diagnosed with Parkinson's Disease. I loved dancing to music. I was surfing the internet and came across MMDG Dance for PD. It made me cry because I was able to find something that I could continue doing what I loved to do [...]. Dance even though I was diagnosed with PD.
>
> I called Mark Morris and found out there was a workshop which I registered for [...]. Everyone went around telling who they were and what they did. It got to me and I always love saying this. My name is Jane McDonald. I come from Cape Cod and I have Parkinson's. I want to teach a class. When I said I have PD they looked over at me and questioned 'How can you teach if you have Parkinson's?' I was the only one there with PD.
>
> The workshop gave me the tools to start a class. One of the things I remember is I was told to teach what you know.
>
> (McDonald 2015)

Risch and Beaton, a professional dance teacher, joined McDonald to co-lead the sessions. Risch not only credits Dance for PD with giving her the skills to teach her programme, but also with giving her 'the tools to find my way back to dance' (Risch 2015). In this instance, Dance for PD motivated the women to set up a class, as well as welcomed a return to dance and work for two women diagnosed with Parkinson's.

The training programme's success lies not just in the meticulous attention given to its content, nor that it facilitates networking, but also in how it has travelled around the world. The programme's ability to travel has given dance teaching artists unable to afford to go to New York the opportunity to experience the training in their own countries and in the process generate more networking and development within that region. It has also meant that experienced Dance for PD teaching artists have been able to undertake continuing professional development in their own countries in order to keep their practice fresh and maintain high-quality delivery.

## Dance for Parkinson's in Britain

### Early UK initiatives

In the seaside town of Weymouth, south-west England, a dance for Parkinson's class takes place. It is called 'the exercise group' and has been subsidized by the Parkinson's UK Dorchester and Weymouth Branch since 2001.[6] The class takes place in an unassuming community room on a social housing estate. The floor is carpeted and high-backed armchairs dominate the space. The teaching artist, Amanda Fogg, uses ideas developed through her experience as a community dance artist and honed through the years working with the Parkinson's group. Most of the participants are men. Their wives sit chatting at the back of the room. The majority are white working class, reflective of the demographic on the estate. Participants stand behind the armchairs, holding on for support while they extend their legs out to the front, pointing and flexing their feet. They dance to recorded music on a CD player. Later, chairs pushed to the side, participants process down the centre of the room, imagining wearing a cloak and crown to develop large, sweeping gestures and an upright posture.

Living in a largely rural area, participants do not have many opportunities to dance or to see live dance performances. Calling it an exercise class was a deliberate attempt on Fogg's part to integrate dancing within a context where dance was not present (Fogg 2010). Fogg herself felt isolated from the dance community when she started the class. As an independent dance teaching artist in a rural location, she did not have many chances to talk about what she was doing. It was only seven years later that she met other dance for Parkinson's teaching artists and was able to start a conversation about her work (Fogg 2010).

One of her first British contacts had founded her own class in 2006 without knowing about Fogg's initiative. Nestled in the Lake District of England, a community hall serves as a venue for the class led by neurophysiotherapist and dance teaching artist, Daphne Cushnie. The hall is situated in the middle of the small town of Kendal. It has a wooden floor, with plastic chairs arranged in a circle for the beginning of class:

> Sitting in a circle, the dance participants unfurl their left arms and, impelled by the twist in the spine, sweep their right arms across their bodies to unite both hands together. Tom then draws the right arm back across his body to the right side through a number of minute articulations of the arm, head and torso. On the other side of the room Charles moves his arm very slowly across his body with great concentration, creating a sense of a special space in between his torso and hand. Meanwhile Oriel's eyes light up as her husband sitting next to her touches her hand and Bella laughs as she realizes she has gone a different way to everyone else.
>
> (Houston field notes, Kendal 2010)[7]

Working mainly with improvised movement, as well as some loosely set material, Cushnie draws out creative ideas within the class, often using props, such as balls and scarves. Like

Fogg, Cushnie uses recorded music. The emphasis is on dynamic alignment and controlled posture too, as well as finding ways to remember the sequences of movement material through tactics such as using imagery to describe movements (Cushnie 2008).

Both Cushnie and Fogg met at the Dance for PD training programme. Fogg attended one of the first Dance for PD training workshops in 2007 to find support and refresh her work (Fogg 2008). She notes that the Dance for PD training gave her the connection that she had been seeking to the wider dance world, as well as inspiration and practical help (Fogg 2010). Yet the Dance for PD training programme did not just aid individual practitioners, such as Fogg and Cushnie, but was a catalyst for the set-up of a national network of teaching artists, the Dance for Parkinson's Partnership UK, that enabled dance for Parkinson's to be embedded within the UK community dance infrastructure.

The beginnings of the UK Partnership can be traced back to 2008 when MMDG performed at Dance Umbrella, the prestigious London-based contemporary dance festival, which, years earlier, had first brought Mark Morris to the attention of British audiences. Toby Beazley, Dance Umbrella's executive director, recognized the potential of the Dance for PD programme for British community dance and asked Leventhal and Heginbotham, both still touring with the company, to lead a workshop whilst they were in London.

For several dance teaching artists, this workshop was the catalyst to begin to teach dance for Parkinson's. For example, the enthusiasm of Joanne Duff, ballet dancer and teaching artist, led to her joining Musical Moving, a small-scale organization offering dance for Parkinson's classes around London, which had been co-founded by musician and dancer Anna Gillespie, dance movement therapist Marina Benini and dance educator Marion North, who had Parkinson's herself. Musical Moving has run a variety of long-lasting and one-off dance sessions within London, most notably in a community health centre in Kentish Town, north London and in a community hall in Wimbledon, south-west London.

Meanwhile, Mo Morgan was inspired to start a class in 2009 at Edinburgh's Dance Base, the organization that caters for community and professional dancers in south-east Scotland. The class was popular, so when Morgan moved to Cornwall, Scottish Ballet took it over to sustain the programme. Gemma Coldicott similarly took on a Parkinson's exercise class in Croydon, south London, in 2008. She recreated it as a creative dance class in content, although maintained its label as an exercise and movement class 'so as not to put off the many men' who attended (Coldicott 2010). Sharing ideas and practices with increasingly experienced teaching artists has cultivated their enthusiasm for the network.

## The Dance for Parkinson's Partnership UK

The 2008 Dance for PD workshop became not just a catalyst for individual dance teaching artists and organizations to develop their own dance for Parkinson's sessions, but for that group of teaching artists and musicians to create their own network to foster sharing of good practice and provide mutual support. The group started to meet two or three times a year from 2011 to share practice, ideas and challenges, and whenever MMDG came to perform in the United Kingdom, the Partnership invited Leventhal to lead a workshop.

From 2013, the UK Partnership began to widen through the establishment of an annual international professional development course. Other teaching artists and organizations, who had their own individual inflections of dance for Parkinson's sessions, joined. For instance, Beatrice Ghezzi, a Limòn specialist, adapted this modern dance technique to suit those with Parkinson's, keeping in the form's characteristic use of weight; Paul MacDonald, a professional clown with Parkinson's, brought his movement skills and Parkinson's experience to a dance programme co-led by contemporary dance artist Natalie Speake; Rebecca Seymour brought expertise in facilitating dance for older people to bear on specific dance for Parkinson's classes; Scottish Ballet brought the experience and understanding gained from many years of community dance outreach work to bear on setting up a Parkinson's dance programme in Glasgow, Aberdeen and developing the work in Edinburgh. Similarly Rambert Dance Company did the same in London, developing its long-term interest in older people dancing. The UK Partnership champions no specific style or form of dance, and embraces social dances, such as the tango, salsa and Irish and English folk dance, too. Many people with Parkinson's join mainstream classes in social dance, rather than one dedicated to dance for Parkinson's. Writing about teaching tango to a mixed group of people with and without Parkinson's in Cambridge, England, Connatty et al. (2013) point out that it is possible for a person with Parkinson's to obtain in-class support and one-to-one tuition in a mainstream class, enabling her or him to comfortably complete a standard beginner's course independently.

The growth of the UK Partnership was facilitated by partnerships with larger organizations, without which the network could not have developed and possibly could not have survived. Such a venture takes time, energy, contacts, management expertise and money, some things that are more easily catered for, or subsumed within, larger organizations than taken on by independent dance teaching artists. First, Dance Umbrella provided the impetus to collect around a common aim, and it helped support workshops through its professional friendship with host venues. It also helped the network successfully apply for two grants to scale up its activity. Second, two universities with dance departments, University of Roehampton, London and De Montfort University, Leicester provided the UK Partnership with space to hold its international professional development courses.[8] Four dance organizations involved with dance for Parkinson's – English National Ballet, Rambert, Scottish Ballet and Pavilion Dance South West – offered to host and organize smaller workshops and meetings.

The professional development courses run by the UK Partnership are crucial regular meeting points for teaching artists working and wanting to work with people with Parkinson's. Taught by experienced dance for Parkinson's teaching artists, they have allowed a body of knowledge to be shared, explored and passed on. The courses have allowed those teaching artists and dance companies working in the community to gain a fundamental understanding of Parkinson's and of good teaching practice in relation to the context. In this way, the professional development courses have been instrumental in growing the pool of teaching artists that can deliver dance for Parkinson's classes, not only around the United Kingdom but also internationally.[9]

Significantly, though, the catalyst for embedding this growth within the arts infrastructure was the partnership established with People Dancing, the national strategic development organization for community and participatory dance in the United Kingdom. In 2013, People Dancing (then known as the Foundation for Community Dance) took on the UK Partnership as one of its specialist practice groups, helped put in place a governance structure in the form of first a steering group and then, once money was in place, a directorship with an advisory group and gave access to its professional development, fundraising and support frameworks. For example, People Dancing took over the administration of the UK Partnership's professional development courses by incorporating them into its high-profile annual summer school, which offered various courses for dance teaching artists. It also established an online training course in conjunction with Dance for PD, to help cement knowledge and understanding about Parkinson's and thereby augment the quality of the face-to-face professional development courses. The online training course is now a prerequisite to participation in the summer school and Dance for PD's training courses in the United States, Canada and Australia. With significant funding from the Baring Foundation, People Dancing recruited a director, Kiki Gale, to bring vision and management to the network and to augment the support and provision of dance for people with Parkinson's.

The United Kingdom presents an interesting case study of an emerging network that has been influenced and inspired by Dance for PD, but also has its own associations and inflections. The UK Partnership is an important example of how independent, often isolated, initiatives can integrate into, and be embraced by, a larger infrastructure and how support for specialist dance provision may grow. This British case study can be considered a success story of the Dance for PD training programme influencing the spread and development of dance for Parkinson's. From a connected handful of artists in 2011, to a network engaging with hundreds in 2015, it has escalated the amount of dance for Parkinson's classes offered around the United Kingdom and, to some extent, the rest of Europe, alongside developing quality of practice.

## English National Ballet: An illustration of sustainable and developmental working practice

Fleur Derbyshire-Fox, engagement director at English National Ballet, was also inspired by the initial Dance for PD workshop that led to the foundation of the UK Partnership. She had been tasked with keeping alive the vision of English National Ballet's founders, Anton Dolin and Alicia Markova, of bringing ballet to as wide an audience as possible. Derbyshire-Fox's role in maintaining this vision was to find ways to engage with local communities, both in London and whilst the company was on tour. For Derbyshire-Fox, this meant not necessarily enticing audiences to watch the shows, but to allow mainstream and communities with no history of engagement with dance the chance to experience ballet. She hosted the Dance for PD workshop at Markova House, the London headquarters of English National Ballet. The workshop was a revelation for Derbyshire-Fox, not least because she could see how a touring dance company could establish a dance for Parkinson's programme based on its repertory. Her motivation led to a pilot series of classes in 2010 and the establishment of the English National Ballet Dance for Parkinson's programme in 2011. The weekly class is taught by specialist dance teaching artists, Danielle Teale (née Jones) and Rebecca Trevitt, and musicians, Jon Petter and Nathan Tinker; they initially were mentored by Anna Gillespie and Joanne Duff of Musical Moving and also completed Dance for PD training in New York. The programme content is inspired by a work or works in the company's current repertory. The movement is based on the principles of ballet (explained below), although not necessarily balletic steps. The music from the repertory is an integral element of the programme and participants engage in voice work as part of their warm up. Voice work is a useful element in warming up the body gently, as well as an accessible way of experimenting with rhythm, expression and communication. The programme also consists of subsidized visits to the theatre to see the company perform, along with talks by wig makers, costume designers, conductors, orchestral musicians and archivists.

English National Ballet took seriously the idea of sustaining and nurturing dance for Parkinson's by using its influence in the British and international dance sector to develop a programme of mentoring and teaching within a group of partners. English National Ballet's initial pilot project of twelve weeks grew into a long-term programme, with classes in London and four British cities to which the company toured – Oxford, Liverpool, Ipswich and Cardiff. Delivery partnerships with local organizations in these cities (Oxford City Council, MDI, DanceEast and National Dance Company Wales) led to the creation of dance for Parkinson's 'hubs' and involved the mentoring of a local dance artist and musician to lead the groups. The delivery partner organizations administered and marketed the programme in each location, with English National Ballet providing the content, strategic direction of the programme and mentoring of the teaching artists. The strong ties between the partners created a close network of people experienced in delivering dance for Parkinson's programmes in several British regions.

In addition to participating in the UK Partnership professional development courses, English National Ballet offered one professional development course through each of the hubs for interested dance teaching artists and musicians in the region. These led to many more teaching artists interested in starting classes. Similar to both the Dance for PD and UK Partnership training programmes, English National Ballet established itself as another base for teacher development. The company offered a different approach, however, maintaining control over its method of teaching through its repertory and creating English National Ballet associate artists in different regions. In addition, it created long-lasting relationships with other organizations to help deliver its way of working. English National Ballet's approach, based on partnership working, additionally offered quality control through appointing English National Ballet associate artists with ongoing sharing of practice amongst the hubs.

Other international dance companies have replicated English National Ballet's way of working, not only in the Dance for PD-inflected mode of delivery, but in inviting researchers to study the benefits of the programmes. An invitation from Queensland Ballet in Australia to English National Ballet's artistic director Tamara Rojo to be a guest performer led to a friendship between Queensland Ballet's Education Department and English National Ballet's Engagement Department. The Australian company was inspired to set up a dance for Parkinson's class using English National Ballet and Dance for PD as guides, and it invited a Dance for PD-certified teacher, Erica Jeffrey, to teach and coordinate the programme. Jeffrey had been working with Leventhal to develop dance for Parkinson's classes in Australia and had instigated the first Dance for PD workshop for teaching artists, led by Leventhal, in Brisbane in 2013. The ballet connection was important to the Australian company in establishing the content of classes and ways of working. Also, following English National Ballet's format, Queensland Ballet commissioned research alongside its artistic programme, using the University of Roehampton's model of mixed-methods research (Jeffrey 2014a), which had allowed English National Ballet to argue for and expand its dance for Parkinson's programme. Commissioning research provided the possibility of advocating, but also it enabled a group of researchers from Queensland University of Technology to contribute to knowledge about dancing with Parkinson's (Lamont et al. 2016). Queensland Ballet developed a successful programme with trips to the theatre for participants and a class based on the company's repertory. Thanks to the efforts of Jeffrey to expand the practice, the growth of dance for Parkinson's classes in Australia was quick, with nineteen classes established between 2013 and 2016 in New South Wales, Victoria, Australian Capital Territory, as well as Queensland (Jeffrey 2014b, 2016).

Hamilton City Ballet in Ontario, Canada, heard about the English National Ballet programme through the Roehampton research study and was inspired to start a class based on the repertory approach. The company also commissioned its own research from McMaster University, led by music cognition scientist Matthew Woolhouse (Woolhouse et al. 2015). Meanwhile, the National Ballet of Canada School, Toronto, set up a Dance for PD class and partnered with local York University on a research project led by neuroscientist Joseph De Souza (Dhami et al. 2015). As part of the school's Sharing the Dance programme, the dance for Parkinson's sessions have led to a potentially interesting intergenerational connection with the young trainee professional dancers. These Canadian examples and that of Queensland Ballet illustrate that dance for Parkinson's research also may become the vehicle for expanding international networks of dance provision.

## European networks and approaches

Dance for Parkinson's networks criss-cross the globe, including those separate from Dance for PD. One network began in the Netherlands. When Marc Vlemmix, the executive director of the Tilburg Dance House, the Netherlands, was diagnosed with Parkinson's at the age of 37, he asked the resident ballet master and choreographer Andrew Greenwood to help him move again. Together they began to experiment with dance, exploring what was useful, invigorating and fun to do (Vlemmix 2014). When the Dance House closed in 2012 because of a shift in the government's arts funding policy, Vlemmix and Greenwood established the foundation Dance for Health in May of the following year. Within eighteen months, Dance for Health had fifteen classes throughout the Netherlands and had trained 22 teaching artists (Greenwood 2014a). As with many other dance for Parkinson's programmes, Dance for Health is passionate about its connection to art and to dancing, rather than seeing its work as therapy (Greenwood 2014b). The Netherlands does not have a tradition of Dance Houses offering community dance as Britain does, and so when the Dutch government changed the focus of its arts funding to encourage more interaction with local communities, Dance for Health reflected this new agenda better than the old Tilburg Dance House. Although offering a theatrical environment with an artistic focus, Dance for Health is more concerned with engaging local Parkinson's communities with dance and other art (for example musical soirées and photography exhibitions), than with creating highly polished dance productions.

Dance for Health's aim is to create a forum where people may be inspired and may change their lives through movement. The philosophy has developed such that the emphasis in the classes has changed from teacher-led to participant-led.

> Greenwood gives the floor to Vlemmix. We all copy him, dancing to 'Say a Prayer' by Enya. We lift our arms above our heads, crossing our wrists, opening our arms out to the side and we lift the backs of our elbows up and then down, leaving the wrists to trail down afterwards like a bird in flight.
>
> (Houston field notes, Bassano del Grappa 2014)

In the class described here, Vlemmix then gave the floor to another participant, and after leading the dance, she gave it to another. Giving the lead to a participant and witnessing and participating in her dance acknowledges the ability of the leader. Some dance organizations including both disabled and non-disabled participants in the United Kingdom use this technique as a cornerstone of their classes.[10] The technique helps celebrate difference and privilege dancers who may feel limited in their ability to respond to set phrases led by a teacher. This creates a subtle shift in power from teacher to participant, breaking down the traditional, hierarchical relationship.

Dance for Health's network extended not only across the Netherlands, but also to Bassano del Grappa, Italy, where a dance for Parkinson's class – Dance Well – was established in the civic museum. Instigated by the director of dance projects for the Centro per la Scena Contemporanea, Roberto Casarotto, in conjunction with Dance for Health, it became a hub for the local community and people with Parkinson's.

> Standing in a room lined with photographs we reach up and twist a 'bunch of grapes', walking round in a small circle to do so. We bring our arms down across our bodies to

the 'bag' at our hip. (We are told that we are unique, that no one is wrong, everyone is right.) We trample the grapes, bringing our knees up and stamp our feet down into the ground. (We are told to love our bodies.) Later on the command of 'cappuccino!' we all raise our arms and lift one leg in the air. I hold onto the hand of a large, bearded man. He has Parkinson's. We smile to each other. This is fun and he's just balanced on one leg.

(Houston field notes, Bassano del Grappa 2014)

Bassano del Grappa is a small, old town near Venice, which hosts an international contemporary arts festival each year. Casarotto met Greenwood and Vlemmix when curating a European dance festival of older people dancing, Act Your Age (2012–13), and asked them to help set up Dance Well. Dance for Health mentored fifteen Italian dance teaching artists, who took monthly turns to lead the weekly dance sessions in Bassano. This approach to working with a range of teaching artists gives dance participants (with and without Parkinson's) experience of different styles and ways of moving, which keeps them exploring new movement pathways. Now independent from Dance for Health, Dance Well is part of the contemporary arts scene in Bassano. Contemporary dance choreographers create dance productions with the group as performers, and through this initiative, the local community may become artists.

Like Dance for PD and English National Ballet's stance of integrating their groups into the dance company's studios, running a dance for Parkinson's class in a museum, as in Bassano del Grappa, is a deliberate attempt to emphasize the artistic nature of the class. In Freiburg, Germany, the Modern Art gallery is also the venue for the dance for Parkinson's class run by Theatre Freiburg from 2013. In the first few months, there was an exhibition by artist Heike Beyer in the gallery next to the dance room consisting of wilting flowers and entitled *Scarcely Able to Stand*. Beyer's intention was to meditate on how forms change through time (RAM publications 2016), and the connection to how Parkinson's changes bodies through time – until people are scarcely able to stand – was not lost on the dance participants. Beyer's work drew out the beauty in the decaying flowers by keeping their heads lifted with long threads. In the same way, the Parkinson's dancers concluded that their dance practice brought out the beauty in their bodies.

In the Freiburg example, the cross-fertilization of ideas from other programmes is evident. The idea of the art gallery hosting the class was directly borrowed from Theatre Freiburg's link with Roberto Casarotto in Bassano. The inclusion of voice work in the sessions was influenced by English National Ballet's class. One of Freiburg's two teaching artists, Monica Gillette, attended the dance for Parkinson's professional development course with English National Ballet in Liverpool. During a class at the Modern Art gallery, Mia Habib, Gillette's teaching partner, led an exercise based on embodying expression and communication after a voice warm-up:

Habib calls out in a squeaky voice; her right arm flutters. It's nonsense, but it sounds like she's saying something to the woman in the blue top across the circle. The woman in the blue top embraces the nonsensical sentence in her body wrapping her arms around herself and then shoots out her arms and legs strongly as she shouts in an angry low voice to the man in grey trousers sitting next to me. He 'jumps' his upper body back as if absorbing the shock of her abuse and sends the verbal instruction to a woman with red lipstick in a high Micky Mouse voice. We all laugh.

(Houston field notes, Freiburg Museum für Neue Kunst 2014)

In this exercise, the expression put into the voice reverberates in the body. It is also a chance to articulate the voice imaginatively and provocatively in ways that adults do not usually do.

Jon Petter, music educationalist and lead musician for the English National Ballet Dance for Parkinson's programme, champions music and voice work as not just an accompaniment to the dancing, but as an equal partner. The musicians are actively involved in the teaching of every English National Ballet class; they are not just accompanists. Gillespie, who first mentored the English National Ballet musicians, explains the importance of vocal exercises:

I have noticed that dancers who are clearly involved with the music often find enhanced ease in accessing movement. This has led me to search for more ways to encourage dancers to develop as deep a connection with music as possible. One of these is the introduction of vocal work to our dance classes. Simple vocal exercises are great for warming up the body, finding breath as a support for movement, and are essentially expressive and fun. Embodying a rhythm or melodic phrase by singing has a very positive impact on movement, which is then performed to the same or similar rhythm played on the piano.

(Gillespie cited in Duff et al. 2011)

Hugo Tham, a dance teaching artist working along the west coast of Sweden, agrees. A former professional ballet dancer and former professional counter-tenor, Tham delivers both dance and technical vocal exercises to people with Parkinson's that reflect his unusual mix of career. He argues that the voice work is a very important part of the Parkinson's dancers' training. Tham (2017) states, '[y]ou don't have to study the consequences of the Parkinson's disease for very long before you come up on the fact that the voice together with the whole breathing system slowly degenerates'. He asserts that the voice is fundamentally connected to the body and that if there is no movement, there is no sound. He gives examples of his voice exercises, which release the voice through movement – '[w]e find sounds inspired by movement that helps us get the power from the big muscles of the back and from the gluteus and thighs' (Tham 2017) – but he is adamant that these exercises are nothing without art-making: 'We paint the room with vast sound movements. We make sound moves, move sounds, – we make movement richer and sound greater' (Tham 2017).

At English National Ballet, voice work also becomes a means of learning more about the music in the company repertory, as well as about some of the metres and rhythmic patterns that will be used in the dance class. For example, the leaders of the English Ballet Dance for Parkinson's programme chose to use the Neapolitan dances from Act 3 of *Swan Lake* (Deane, after Petipa and Ivanov, 1997). Fast and intricate, the piece of music was deliberately chosen as a seated rhythmic exercise. Clapping out separate rhythms to the chanting of 'piz-za', 'mar-ga-ri-ta', 'fior-en-ti-na' and 'na-poli-ta-na', the class divided into pizza slices to create a complex layering of sound while the music was played at the same time on the piano. This exercise developed into a movement exercise staying with the theme of ordering in a pizza restaurant but with the rhythms still evident in the timing of the movement. It became a fun and slightly irreverent way of relating to a well-known, exuberant and rhythmically intricate section in *Swan Lake*.

## Approaches to teaching and values of practice

A widely copied version of structuring a dance for Parkinson's class is the one offered by Dance for PD, which was embraced by English National Ballet.

The classes start seated to emphasize the inclusion of all, even those who may feel unsteady, or are not able to stand. The circular formation, important in much community dance, stresses this idea of inclusion, of witnessing and acknowledging each other, emphasizing that they dance as a group. Although a circle might feel exposing, most Parkinson's participants and teaching artists see it as a welcoming space. Additionally, warming up the body and the mind while seated gives participants the ability to start dancing without worrying about falling over.

The content of the sessions is highly individual, based on the creativity and dance traditions of the teaching artists and the contributions of the individual participants. The English National Ballet class (attended by approximately 40 participants at any one time in London) is an inclusive dance class based on the principles of ballet and with movement differentiation. Movement is adapted or created differently for individuals in the group who have differing needs and physical abilities. As noted above, the music is from English National Ballet's repertoire, including works such as *The Rite of Spring* (MacMillan/Stravinsky, 1962), *In the Middle Somewhat Elevated* (Forsythe/Willems, 1987) and *The Nutcracker* (Eagling/Tchaikovsky, 2010). Improvisation is included within the sessions. As with the Dance for PD sessions, the class starts seated, progresses to standing and then to moving across the studio. Although ballet 'steps' are not necessarily used (the arabesque, the pirouette), there is an emphasis on lengthening the spine and limbs, projecting energy through eye focus and an enlarged kinesphere, and changing dynamics and qualities of movement. Despite working within the ballet oeuvre, the sessions are not concerned with constricting the movement vocabulary to the ballet lexicon, or with how movements are executed. Indeed, individual ways of moving are celebrated. The two musicians, Petter and Tinker, improvise around the ballet's score, and the improvisatory approach to music mirrors the open attitude to the movement. The teaching artists lead through a person-centred approach, focusing the class on the abilities people have, and acknowledging and witnessing individual contributions.

A strong focus within the Dance for PD training programme, as well as the English National Ballet programme, is an emphasis on the values and principles by which the teaching artists work. As noted above, Dance for PD argues that the class is about dancing and participants are treated as dancers. It is telling that in the film *Capturing Grace* (Iverson 2014a), one participant, Reggie, pronounces: 'There are no patients. There are only dancers'. Parkinson's might bring people to the studio, but once they are there, Parkinson's is not the primary focus. As White notes, '[a]rts activity enables a search for meaning and value by and for the whole person and not just for the sick or dysfunctional part' (White 2009: 4–5). This principle is complemented by core values based on mutual respect, inclusiveness, enjoyment, community, collaboration, creativity, innovation and artistic excellence (Dance for PD 2011).

The two values of respect and inclusiveness are demonstrated through particular ways of facilitating the class. They are key components of many community dance initiatives that work to include people with diverse needs and abilities, although specific teaching techniques and ideas on what inclusion means may vary from teaching artist to teaching artist. Dance scholar Christina Kostoula (2012) points out that teaching artists cannot be complacent when devising dance sessions for those whose movement, or ability to synthesize movement, might be compromised. Whichever method of including diversity is used within the dance class, Kostoula explains, '[a]n inclusive manner means that we prepare and organize a class so that the presence (or not) of a different body will not pose problems to the ethos and the purpose of the lesson' (2012: 81). In other words, in valuing inclusivity, the teaching artist or dance organization has to find ways of bringing everybody into the session so that each person can participate and experience dance as an art form.

Dance for PD and English National Ballet, both of whom largely use a method where the teaching artist invents a sequence of movements to be loosely copied by the dancers, use techniques of differentiation and adaptation: the teaching artist is clear in showing participants what to do to perform an exercise in different ways, according to how they are feeling, or their ability on a particular day. For example, standing work might incorporate a seated version for a person who is feeling particularly vulnerable to falling over. These adaptations are then encouraged in an open and flexible manner, often with an assistant or another teaching artist giving individual attention to the particular dancer who requires an adapted exercise, or with one teaching artist dancing the adaptation, whilst another dances the original version, allowing participants to choose. In tandem, the inclusion of much participant-led improvisation in exercises allows for the material to be dictated by the skill and abilities of the participants. These are both witnessed and given prominence within the session.

## Issues facing dance for Parkinson's teaching artists

Although the dance for Parkinson's global network is successfully growing and many dance teaching artists are enhancing their understanding of how to facilitate classes for people with Parkinson's, many issues affect the development of dance for Parkinson's as a major specialist dance practice. Funding classes is a major issue. Many dance for Parkinson's teaching artists believe that participants should not need to pay much, if at all for classes. Typically, people with Parkinson's do not work and have fixed household incomes. Those living in countries where healthcare is not free at point of delivery have to spend increasing amounts of money on medication and other forms of healthcare. Teaching artists recognize the importance of accessibility of classes, and many attempt to gain subsidy or a grant to reimburse them for teaching the classes, or they charge a small amount to try to cover costs. Payment for class is usually minimal, and this can contribute to the problem of sustaining the class.

Many teaching artists spend much time writing funding applications to elicit more subsidy for the class, but as Leventhal notes, dance for Parkinson's falls between two types of funding:

Funding is always a battle. It's a challenge as it's a hybrid programme. The emphasis is on arts based classes, but there's definitely a health care component. People who fund healthcare programmes often are not interested in funding arts organisations. Conversely many arts organisations think of it not as arts, so you're trapped in limbo. Funders who get it, get it, or have missions which are both arts and health.

(Leventhal 2010)

Large- and medium-scale dance companies usually are more successful in gaining funding than most independent artists. They may have development offices that can apply for funds on behalf of the programme, or they may be able to fund their classes through core budget activities, creating a financial buffer at least in the short term.

Many independent teaching artists have established relationships with local Parkinson's support groups, which support their dance classes. Obtaining funding from other sources, such as trusts and foundations, or through arts funding schemes, is harder for independent teaching artists, not least because many lack skills in fundraising. Working voluntarily on a time-consuming application also can be demoralizing if many are unsuccessful.

Dance for Parkinson's classes also can be time consuming to run, and the lead teaching artists often need assistants to help keep classes as safe as they can be for individual participants. Tango teacher Anna Leatherdale points out that paying a support worker means that the 'sessions are completely uneconomical' (Leatherdale 2013). Musical Moving teacher Joanne Duff notes that most of the work, carried out by her and other teaching artists, happens on a voluntary basis (Duff 2013). This is a problem as it means that classes are vulnerable to being closed, if the teaching artist cannot cope financially or emotionally with the unpaid effort given to the classes. Joanie Carlisle from Dixon, New Mexico, United States, attended the Dance for PD training programme in 2011 in order to develop her existing practice and address a challenge: making a living from it. She runs classes in Dixon and Albuquerque, more than two hours away, and at that time, the income from the classes did not cover the period she spent preparing for, driving to and teaching the classes. Carlisle gets the space for free, but as each group has different needs, she must organize different music and material. Being paid a decent wage to facilitate classes is one of the issues that must be addressed for the professionalization of the dance teaching artist. Many teaching artists, like Carlisle, keep their classes going because they have a vocation and passion for the work. They feel a responsibility to maintain a class that participants find important to their state of well-being.

Emotional toll for dance for Parkinson's teaching artists is high and this is a major issue. Teaching artist Rachel Canavan explains:

> When people are faced with such physical challenges, it is difficult to detach yourself from the raw emotion of this physical loss. Dancers value movement in different ways than most people, the body is their instrument. So when you value movement so greatly, you have natural compassion for these physical challenges participants face when they dance.
> (Canavan 2013)

The UK Partnership allows teaching artists working with people living with Parkinson's in Britain to air these issues and share experiences of dealing with them, and the advanced teacher training courses run by Dance for Parkinson's Australia include sessions on how to deal with bereavement. The wider Dance for PD network also provides an outlet for sharing common challenges, which is particularly useful for the teaching artist who may be the sole practitioner in his or her country. For example, Vonita Singh, working alone in Dubai, cites the encouragement from Dance for PD as helping her find a means to break down barriers and combat social attitudes. Parkinson's is considered shameful in the United Arab Emirates: people with Parkinson's 'are kept behind closed doors' (Singh 2014). Singh hopes to change the culture of shame by using dance in schools to make young people aware of Parkinson's.

Dance teaching artists who specialize in dance for Parkinson's do this work because they are passionate about its benefits and in contributing through dance to a person's quality of life. Despite the issues that they face, they believe that the work is important. Each year at the World Parkinson Coalition's Congress, The People's Choice Award is given to a film that 'captures, inspires and moves hearts', as chosen by people with Parkinson's. The 2016 shortlist featured several films about dancing, selected not only to inspire through endeavour, but particularly because they advocated an alternative, positive lifestyle with Parkinson's. These strategies situate dance for Parkinson's as an artistic enterprise with a social imperative. The message is clear: dancing is one activity that can help project a positive image of people living with Parkinson's. As such, dance may aid in dispelling misunderstandings about the condition and be a constructive way for people affected to relate to Parkinson's. The positive lifestyle conveyed by dance is one reason for why dancing is useful, perhaps even important. Chapter 3 will explore further the question of why dance might be thought of as special.

## Notes

1 Another example is Daniele Volpe, consultant in neurorehabilitation in Vicenza, Italy and amateur Irish folk musician. His interest in researching dance for Parkinson's began when he noted people with Parkinson's coming out of an Irish folk dance club without the habitual symptoms. He also now helps organize dances for people with Parkinson's at his hospital and collaborates with the nearby Dance Well group in Bassano del Grappa.

2   This is not to say that a benefits-driven arts practice is also one propelled by monetary gain, but that both types of practice theoretically may fit into the description of a commodified arts culture.

3   For example, Arts Council England, the body for public funds for the arts in England, has various goals that it asks applicants to address, which are all connected to social relevance. Between 2010 and 2020, the goals included addressing children and young people, addressing diversity and skills and addressing the notion that everyone may have the opportunity to experience art (Arts Council England 2017).

4   The word 'participatory dance' is not used in the same way as the term 'participatory arts', which is part of the visual arts movement engaging with non-trained artists and has more in common with the tradition of cultural democracy. Another general arts term used in the same way is 'socially engaged art', which community dance sometimes appropriates, particularly in the United States (Bishop 2012).

5   The distinction between community arts and health practice and arts therapy is often blurred, but there are differences concerning clinical practice that uses art to develop a patient's health and/or well-being and artistic practice that engages with people with and without illness. Set within a clinical framework, dance movement therapy and dance movement psychotherapy aim to use creative movement to help emotional, social, physical, spiritual and cognitive integration of the self (Association of Dance Movement Psychotherapy 2015) and therapists have gone through extensive, certified training. For dance movement therapy Parkinson's case studies see, for example, Bunce (2002) and Westbrook and McKibben (1989).

6   Parkinson's UK, the largest charity supporting people with Parkinson's and research, works by funding local branches (groups of people living with Parkinson's in a specific geographical location) to promote activity within local areas.

7   This description is published in *Dance Research* by Edinburgh University Press (Houston 2011: 330).

8   The University of Roehampton through my association with the UK Partnership and De Montfort University through its association with People Dancing.

9   For example, two Swedish dance teaching artists attended the 2014 summer school and then instigated a Swedish network of independent dance teaching artists interested in dance for Parkinson's in 2015.

10  AMICI Dance Theatre champions this way of working, for example, because of the wide range of physical and mental abilities represented by company members.

## Chapter 3

What's so special about dancing?

A t the end of Chapter 2, I suggested that the positivity that dancing engenders is useful and perhaps even important to people with Parkinson's. This chapter tackles the broader question about the specialness of dancing by providing several arguments for the consideration of why it might be important. With several activities that have claims to be therapeutic for people with Parkinson's (see for example, Gao et al. 2014; Snijders and Bloem 2010), clarifying what is special about dancing explains why we should pay it attention. Furthermore, interrogating specialness allows for a critical examination of the claims of benefit and distinctiveness made by the dance sector and participants. The arguments are not exhaustive, but are ones that have surfaced within dance for Parkinson's research and practice and so are particularly relevant to the context. The chapter takes in arguments that are evidence-based and also those that are tied to people's subjective experiences of dancing with Parkinson's. It lays out arguments for physical benefit, as well as for the importance of specific elements within dance, such as music, movement learning and recall strategies, and aesthetic elements, such as the body's relationship to time and space (a peculiarly pertinent topic for people with Parkinson's), movement qualities and dynamics. This chapter highlights what is special about dancing that distinguishes this art form from other kinds of physical exercise. It describes the evidence for physical and other benefits, as well as arguing for elements of dance that promote feelings of health and well-being.

## Use it or lose it

One of the primary aspects of dancing is that it moves and exercises the body in various ways and to various degrees depending on the dance form. Dancing is seen as a fun way – and therefore an easier way – to keep fit and healthy. People with Parkinson's are not excluded from this and evidence suggests that exercise helps control several Parkinson's symptoms (Nieuwboer 2009). The evidence shows that, in general, people in western societies do not do enough physical activity (British Heart Foundation National Centre for Physical Activity and Health 2009). The Health Survey for England (HSCIC 2012), which monitored trends in physical activity and inactivity across the country, found that 74 per cent of men and 76 per cent of women over age 85 do not participate in the recommended amount of physical activity for that age group. Surveys reveal that around 40 per cent of men aged between 65 and 85 are not physically active despite knowing the possible consequences (HSCIC 2012; Thurston and Green 2004). Using different data, Skelton and colleagues (1999) reported that in 1999, only 20 per cent of British adults over 50 were walking briskly five days a week.

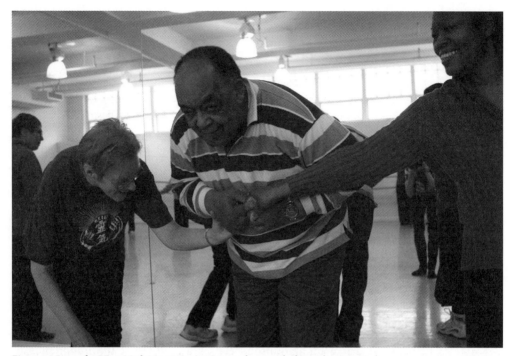

**Figure 3:** Dance for PD at Mark Morris Dance Center, photography by Amber Star Merkens.

Yet, many highly publicized research studies point out that physical inactivity is one of the easiest factors to modify in order to achieve better health (World Health Organization 2007; Farrell et al. 2014; Scarborough et al. 2011). Given that the prospect of maintaining regular physical activity is low in the general population (Farrell et al. 2014), the World Health Organization (2007) recommends that physical activity be integrated easily into people's lives. Researching adherence to exercise in later life, Miranda Thurston and Ken Green found that in order for people to commit to regular exercise, 'richness in terms of satisfactions and skills generated through particular activities' encourages commitment to regular exercise (2004: 383). In addition, tailoring exercise to people's needs produces better results (Riddoch et al. 1998; Thurston and Green 2004; British Heart Foundation National Centre for Physical Activity and Health 2009; Connolly and Redding 2010).

Several evidence-based reviews report that taking up physical activity becomes more important as people age because of their increased risks of falling, chronic disease and mortality (World Health Organization 2007: 6; Public Health England 2014; HSCIC 2012). An international systematic review of the literature in 2010 on the cost of falls estimated that falls in people over 65 living in the community cost 23.3 billion US dollars in the United States and the equivalent of 1.6 billion US dollars in the United Kingdom (Davis et al. 2010). In a partnership study between researchers and 1000 people living with Parkinson's in the

United Kingdom, balance and falls topped the list of ten priorities for research into the management of Parkinson's (Deane et al. 2014).[1] As fall risk is extremely high for people with Parkinson's, it becomes important to find a form of exercise that challenges stability, thereby leading to improved ability to prevent falling.

Dance for people over 50 is seen as an effective way of exercising because it can be tailored to people's requirements and is a sociable way of learning new skills (Connolly and Redding 2010; Keogh et al. 2009). In other words, dance can fit into people's lifestyles relatively easily and can be an accessible form of exercise. Connolly and Redding (2010) point to dance's ability to incorporate multiple modes of exercise, such as aerobic and anaerobic training, strength, flexibility and balance tasks, which are appropriate for older people's needs. This observation is backed up by several studies measuring the impact of exercise on older people in China, Italy and Turkey (Hui et al. 2009; Federici et al. 2005; Eyigor et al. 2009). In terms of fall risk, Federici et al. (2005) and Keogh and colleagues (2009) found in particular that dancing challenges stability by continually shifting the body's centre of gravity away from its base of support, in multiple directions. To regain balance after being taken off-balance requires joint mobility, flexibility, coordination and core strength. Researchers, such as Rehfeld and colleagues (2017) emphasize the ability of dancing to challenge and improve stability to highlight its potential to counteract the risk of falling. Dancing may train the body to regain balance. One consequence of this is not only to lessen the number of falls, but also their consequences, such as hospital stays and disability.

Many participants in dance for Parkinson's classes are aware of the importance of maintaining or developing fitness:

> I thought, ballet, blimey! I'll see how we go. I'm not a great dancer. I'm not disciplined at exercising [...]. This is a discipline. I need to get the weight down. I feel fitter when I'm 3–4 lbs lighter [...]. I do Pilates once a month when I go to the [Parkinson's support] group and someone comes in. But three-quarters of an hour a month is not good enough. I probably should go to the gym [...] but again, I'm not disciplined.
>
> (Roy K 2010)

Many initially saw dancing as an enjoyable and easy way of keeping fit, citing the problem of motivating themselves to exercise on their own:

> I've a lazy mind. I wouldn't do exercise on my own. I'll go anywhere there's a group to make you move [...]. I chose dance because of the movement and it's nice. Gets the muscles moving [...]. Parkinson's is trying to take the muscles so you have to fight back. I want to keep dancing as if you don't use it, you lose it.
>
> (Clare N 2010)

One struggle many older people with Parkinson's have is contending with co-morbidities, such as diabetes, arthritis, even cancer. These may impose their own physical limitations, add to the amount of medication people have to take on a daily basis and potentially contribute to a greater number of stays in hospital. Researchers have found that physical activity helps prevent some of the major chronic diseases, such as heart disease and diabetes, and reduces premature death (Warburton et al. 2006).

Animal and human research also suggests that exercise might be crucial in improving motor function of those with Parkinson's through enabling neuroplasticity (Petzinger et al. 2013). Exercise might aid the brain to create new pathways, bypassing the diseased areas, and to learn how to compensate for any dopamine deficit. These new pathways might enable people to continue to carry out some everyday activities without much difficulty, despite losing dopamine cells.

Although dance for Parkinson's is offered as an artistic activity, rather than as a form of therapy, as discussed in Chapter 2, the majority of the research into the effect of dance on people with Parkinson's has focused on its potential rehabilitative properties, particularly to improve mobility and balance function. Since 1989, when Beth Kaplan Westbrook and Helen McKibben published their controlled study of the neurological and emotional effects of dance movement therapy on groups of outpatients with Parkinson's, there has been a small output of research, notably increasing since 2007. Madeleine Hackney and Gammon Earhart, in particular, contributed to this output in the early days with a number of controlled and comparative research projects and case studies examining tango as a means to promote increased functional mobility, balance and stability in Parkinson's patients. In each study conducted, Hackney and Earhart concluded that dancing the tango over several weeks improved measures in fall risk, gait and balance confidence and facilitated positive social interaction. In comparison to non-dance exercise, results persistently showed that participants who performed tango improved the most (Hackney and Earhart 2009, 2010). Other early research studies examining other dance styles for one month to a year produced similar results using similar research methods. (For examples of some of the first research articles on dance and Parkinson's, see Batson 2010; Heiberger et al. 2011; Houston and McGill 2013; Volpe et al. 2013; Westheimer et al. 2015.) These studies examined a range of styles, such as modern dance, ballet and Irish step dance. All were small-scale investigations, so limited in their findings, but all pointed to the same conclusion: dancing seemed to be good for mobilizing Parkinsonian bodies.

Research into dance for Parkinson's, itself a young practice, gives indications that dancing might not only be a useful way of exercising, but also possibly an effective way of helping control – at least in the short term – some of the motor challenges that people with Parkinson's often possess.

## Learning and recalling

Performing actions is often difficult for people with Parkinson's because their ability to do things at an automatic or subconscious level is impaired (Wu and Hallett 2005). Moreover, since many actions require doing more than one task at any given moment – picking up a cup of tea, walking with it over to a chair and sitting down – impaired ability to process movements automatically makes multitasking difficult (Wu and Hallett 2005; Brown and Marsden 1991). An example of a simple act, which requires multitasking, is picking up a cup of tea from a seated position and drinking it in the company of a friend. This act requires the body to shift forward in the hips (which may mean adjusting feet, lower legs, thighs, bottom, as well as the back), whilst stretching out the arm (which involves activating the muscles in the shoulder girdle and back, a shift in the elbow and shoulder to move forward to stretch), then the opening out of the fingers to slip them between the handle and the body of the cup to clasp the handle, perhaps whilst talking or listening to a friend, then shifting back into the chair (which again involves moving the hips and back, as well as possibly feet, legs and bottom), at the same time as lifting the elbow and hand with the cup to the mouth, whereby the lips need to pucker over the lip of the cup, the jaw to move forward slightly as the head tips back a bit to take a sip, but being careful to adjust the intake to the intensity of heat, whilst still keeping an eye on the friend and listening. This description has missed out the initial intention and feeling of wanting to sip the tea in the first place, whilst talking to the friend and judging the taste of the tea as it slips down the throat. Most of this comes automatically to people, but if one's capacity for voluntary movement is impaired, the simple act of drinking tea may become more difficult. Research has shown, however, that through concentrated practice, people with Parkinson's are able to carry out tasks – such as foot tapping, or counting whilst doing another task – with improved success of completion and at a faster pace (Brown and Marsden 1991; Soliveri et al. 1992; Platz et al. 1998; Wu and Hallett 2005). This research suggests that early- to mid-stage Parkinson's does not destroy people's learning capacities, and that with practice, they may perform tasks with competence.

Learning strategies and techniques for more efficient and stable movement were seen within the pilot research study conducted with English National Ballet's London class (Houston and McGill 2013). Comments by participants, together with the research tasks[2] completed differently by them at the end of twelve weeks of dancing, suggested that participants had increased body awareness and a greater sense of *how* to move with more stability. By the end of the project, many participants could demonstrate various dynamics in movement and change their stance; some could alter their posture. This implies a general increase in awareness of what their body was doing at any given moment. Learning how to do specific actions adds to this awareness, as Mike A (2011) commented: 'I'm using the stick less and less now in the last few weeks. To get up from the chair I've learnt nose over toes'. The balance tasks in the study required volunteers to maintain balance on one leg, to jump safely and to re-stabilize after being knocked off balance. In order to do these tasks successfully, body awareness is required. One participant commented:

Walking on the line and standing on one leg were difficult but improved a lot after the class, but this was in part due to learning the best technique as much as any inherent improvement due to the class. Will try again next week.

(Anon. 1 2010)

This participant places equal emphasis on awareness and physical conditioning for the successful completion of the tasks.

Dancing, formally constituted within specific taught classes, traditionally repeats sequences of movement many times within one session, and over many weeks. This gives participants time to practice tasks and multitasking. In the English National Ballet's London class, participants learnt a sequence of movement for the arms, a *port de bras*, inspired by a scene in *Dust* (2014), a dance work by the British-Bangladeshi choreographer Akram Khan. The seated sequence involved moving arms individually as well as both together through different pathways on horizontal, vertical and sagittal planes.[3] Dancers were encouraged to move their heads in specific directions at the same time, often to follow the moving arm, and they were instructed to bend their torso forward, to the side or backwards at various points. In addition, each movement was specifically timed to create phrasing and dynamics in conversation with a piece of music based on the complicated rhythms of the Japanese Kodo drums. Participants were encouraged to chant a poem that matched the rhythms at the same time as dancing.

The sequence was taught gradually over several weeks, broken down into sections, attempted slowly and then at tempo. Often each movement was described and practised on its own and then in relation to the next movement in the musical phrase. Preparation to familiarize participants with the rhythm of the music involved clapping exercises and chanting the poem, the words of which recalled the intention of the movements. To aid memory of the sequence, the teaching artists invented images evoking the movement rather than giving a mechanical description. The theme of the drumming section in *Dust* was women's work in the First World War in the factories and the home. The images conjured up were pulleys and levers in the factory and tasks, such as stirring a pot, lifting a baby, smoothing out a bed sheet. The contrast in dynamic and quality of movement in the arms was sought with the different images.

The use of familiar images helps with remembering the sequence. For example, Jim S from the English National Ballet's Oxford class recalls in his diary a sequence based on two scenes from Act III of the ballet *The Sleeping Beauty* (Petipa, 1890):

> Thank goodness my ability to follow the routines was much better this week. […] I will try to recall the routine that was based on the handsome prince on horseback: climb on the horse; trot; lasso; bow and arrow; swords; stretch back with hand behind head. There was also a new routine based on Little Red Riding Hood which involved alternating roles of LRRH and the wolf. Preparatory work for this included a fun session led by Jon [Petter, English National Ballet musician] on clapping to a 6/8 rhythm.
>
> (Jim S 2013)

Here the narrative sequence of events helped Jim S remember the movement, although imagery can be used in seemingly abstract sequences too, as seen in the factory images in *Dust*. While these methods of learning are standard practice within a taught dance session, they have the additional benefit of allowing Parkinson dancers to practice and develop motor learning whilst multitasking and to complete motor tasks.

## Moving to music

Several studies have examined how gait (the way people walk) changes for people with Parkinson's in reaction to an outside stimulus, such as a metronome or music (see, for example, McIntosh et al. 1997; Pacchetti et al. 2000; Howe et al. 2003; de Bruin et al. 2010; de Dreu et al. 2012, 2014). These studies suggest that a regular pulse facilitates ease of movement, leading to a faster step cadence and more regular length of stride. More fluid movement whilst dancing has been observed in many dance and other observational studies (Houston and McGill 2011, 2013, 2015; Hackney et al. 2007; Hackney and Earhart 2009; Sacks 2007). The research studies suggest that an external cue, such as music, may give people with Parkinson's an impulse to initiate movement – and in a rhythmic manner – thereby overcoming the challenge of starting movement voluntarily, and creating a regular pulse for stable, rhythmic movement. Some studies also conclude that the effects of the musical pulse stay with people for a short while after the external stimulation has ended (Houston and McGill 2013; Hackney et al. 2007; Hackney and Earhart 2009; Hausdorff et al. 2007; McIntosh et al. 1997).[4]

Dance participants themselves recognize that they have a more fluent or stable walk from dancing. Houston and McGill (2011) reported that one man's increased fluidity in walking meant that he forgot his walking stick after class and set off down the road without it. Pat K writes in her diary:

> Something wonderful is beginning to happen. After I have done my walk, I usually turn around and watch the others as they walk down the diagonal towards the end where I'm standing and what I see is really moving – most of the class are walking to the music with real fluency, including several who I have never seen walk fluently in normal life.
>
> (Pat K 2011)

The diary entries highlight not just the infrequency of fluent walking in everyday life, but also how the ability of participants to regulate walking during the dance session elicits strong emotional reactions.

Fluidity of movement creates a condition for better dynamic stability, where the person is able to come back on balance easily after being destabilized. The research of Michael Hove and colleagues (2012) suggests that stable internal rhythms are vital for the person's own walking patterns. Since people with Parkinson's have less stable internal rhythms, walking patterns are irregular and less steady. Following on from studies comparing walking in healthy participants and those with Parkinson's (Hausdorff et al. 1996; Delignières and Torre 2007; Hausdorff 2009),[5] Hove and colleagues discovered that an external pulse that interacted and changed in response to a person's own walking pattern elicited more stable stride times, a more regular walk with similar strides. This finding is in line with the research into moving to music and Parkinson's. The interaction, however, between external and internal pulses produced more stable stride times than a fixed external pulse on its own. Hove's conclusion was that, although an external pulse can be beneficial for those with Parkinson's, it does not provide the 'flexibility and responsiveness to environmental demands' (Hove et al. 2012: 2731) that an interactive, flexible tempo does, thereby limiting its usefulness. One might surmise, therefore, that dance for Parkinson's classes that are able to hire an experienced musician to accompany a class, rather than relying on recorded music, may replicate this interaction. Dance for Parkinson's musician and teaching artist Anna Gillespie comments on her relationship as a musician to her dancers:

> The sounds and silences that comprise music only become meaningful when an active mind is attending to them and this applies to both dancer and accompanist. It is through this shared, reciprocal and yet personal experience that my musical meeting with dancers occurs. A class never sounds exactly the same because we are all constantly responding to each other. This is particularly useful in a Parkinson's dance class. I'm free to 'personalise' moments in the music, following and/or encouraging the movement of a particular dancer. I can change tempo and quality at will, shifting the 'sense of motion', or try to oblige requests.
>
> (Gillespie cited in Duff et al. 2011)

The 'sense of motion' Gillespie mentions is an interesting way of conceiving of an organic, meaningful dialogue between dancer and musician, between the movement and the music, unlike the unyielding pulse of the metronome. In the hands of an experienced accompanist, music can be a flexible instrument for Parkinson's dancers, changing tempo and rhythm, mood and pulse. In combination with dancing, music may also develop a more physically confident, personal and creative response to movement.

In addition, dance is the opportunity to move in time with others, which can also be beneficial. Sacks ([1973] 1990) found that with an external cue – in this case, chalked lines on the ground – his patient, Miss D, walked with more stability but that her walk was robotic. When Sacks took her by the arm, she responded by walking with fluidity. Dancing with others may provide the opportunity for responding to the rhythms of others (Vicary et al. 2017). The flexible, organic pulse that Hove and colleagues propound may be nurtured in the dancing to live music and in the company of others. Research into synchronization of movement also indicates that it may help direct the movers' attentions to each other and subsequently form better social bonding (Woolhouse et al. 2016).

In some dance for Parkinson's sessions, music is not used to provide tempo, pulse or rhythm – that is, to structure the movement phrases – but to provide a mood, or atmosphere. This means that the pulse that grounds much music and which helps with external cueing for people with Parkinson's is not there, or is not used. Yet some teaching artists who work with music in this way try to stimulate an internal sense of rhythm instead. For example, Lauren Potter, an experienced British contemporary dance performer and teacher, utilizes breath and body weight to structure movement, so that music becomes a way of stating the intention or theme of the movement, or to create an atmosphere. Whether teaching professional dancers or community dancers with Parkinson's, Potter encourages participants to explore their use of breath when moving – so, for example, exploring how breathing out might help the back to twist and how the breathing pattern may induce a flow and rhythm to the subsequent steps – and to sense the weightiness of body parts to carry forward momentum and flow of movement. She encourages people to move more efficiently by first, sensing and imagining the skeletal frame of the body and how the bones (rather than the muscles) might move, second, creating imagery to stimulate the sensing and imagining and third, improvisation to encourage exploration of personal architecture and movement pathways. Moving without recourse to a fixed pulse also has had the observed effect of giving some participants more stability and regularity of movement. For instance, after working in a similar way to Potter with the choreographer Itamar Serussi Sahar, Parkinson's dancer Marc Vlemmix argues that if he just follows the teacher's movements (and so has two outside cues, the music and the teacher) he finds it more difficult to replicate at home. Whereas if he is improvising using his own weight and breath to structure what he is doing, he finds it much easier to utilize this method of moving away from the dance studio than the set phrases of the teacher (Vlemmix 2017). Dancers in Potter's classes and Vlemmix with Serussi Sahar have been guided into finding an inner groundedness and pulse through attention to feeling how the body is working (or getting stuck).

## Exploring space through time

Normally dancing is made up of a series of dynamically enhanced movements, carried out within specific time frameworks. It is also performed with a conscious exploration of the space around the moving body. As pointed out in Chapter 1, people with Parkinson's often experience space differently. Sacks ([1973] 1990) identified challenges related to scale and proprioception: smaller, faster or slower movements are often produced without conscious intention. Other scientists also have noted the problem of impaired proprioception (Adamovich et al. 2001; Jacobs and Horak 2006). Parkinson's causes people to be less aware of where their moving body is in space. Dance may address these problems through encouraging the deliberate amplification or contraction of movement, not only through creating tempo-specific exercises that encourage extension of limbs and eye line and expansion of actions within space, but also by practising precise movements – big and small – that use different dynamic qualities.

Various movement methods encourage the amplification of space for people with Parkinson's. The BIG method, for example, is taken from Lee Silverman's Voice Training (LSVT) method to increase amplification of the voice. BIG aims to enlarge movement specifically to combat the unintended contraction of the kinesphere of people with Parkinson's, that is their relation to the space surrounding their bodies (Ebersbach et al. 2010). The difference between the LSVT BIG method and dance is that dancing encourages increasing accuracy of placement and precise focusing of movement in space, rather than simply more amplification.

Dancing is more than a tool to correct Parkinsonian symptoms. Dance also explores the *aesthetic* potential of movement through space in time. Dance philosopher Sondra Horton Fraleigh (1987) notes the ability of dance to carve through and manipulate space. Stroking, punching, flicking, stamping, bending, drawing, flying the body through space: these actions mould an imaginative canvas on which spatial-temporal narratives are created. The relationship of movement through space is inextricably linked to movement through time. It is impossible to have one without the other. On the whole, this relationship goes unremarked in everyday life, but when dancing, the performer consciously manipulates time and space aesthetically, drawing on a rich palette of dynamics and imagery. The aesthetic and conscious manipulation of time and space allows people with Parkinson's to explore movement that is non-Parkinsonian and pushes against boundaries of habit. For example,

> We are seated in the large studio in Brooklyn where the Mark Morris Dance Group rehearse. We lift one of our arms and imagine we have a paint brush. As the pianist begins to play a medley of Broadway tunes, we write our names on a large imaginary canvas in the air. We convey different colours with contrasting strokes of the arm, some movements stabbing, some languid. We give our other hand a paintbrush too. As the music changes tempo and dynamic, we also vary our movement to complement or counter the music. At one point, my neighbour executes a flourish on my canvas and I on hers. Our painting dance begins to blend into each other's.
>
> (Houston field notes, Dance for PD, Mark Morris Dance Center 2011)

As part of the creation of purposeful, dynamic movement, the dancer develops relationships between his or her body and those of others. In shifting space intentionally through moving (and even through being still), the dancer not only alters space, but forms a dialogue with other bodies occupying the same space.

We interpret human relations and identities through the space they occupy.[6] Thus, the experience of space is personal and subjective. It is not neutral, as dance studies scholar Valerie Briginshaw points out, it 'cannot be explored without reference to human subjects' (2009: 4). For people with Parkinson's in everyday life, this space is often squeezed both physically and symbolically, through a regressing kinesphere, increasing social isolation from others, and the labels 'disabled' and 'non-functioning'. As Parkinson's progresses, both space and relation to oneself and one's identity can alter. Later chapters discuss the potential for dance to create different identities through the aesthetic use of space. What is interesting here is to examine dance's role in reorientating their physical relationship to space and time.

When moving in everyday life, we use our senses to help us judge our environment, where the side of the curb is, where the grass meets the pavement. We typically do not need to look down when moving from the pavement to the grass. Our proprioception judges this movement so that our feet are able to adjust immediately to the difference in texture. When walking down a corridor with an open door half way, we do not think twice about continuing to walk through the doorway and on to the next section of the corridor. Perhaps we might remark that the light is dimmer in this section. When a young child runs across our path, we are able to quickly sense the change to our environment and adjust our gait to avoid colliding with the moving body. We continue our ambulation without a second thought. Our bodies act in relation and subconsciously to their environment in good time to act well. We do not fall over onto the grass, stumble in the dimmed light or bump into the child. Our reactions in and to the physical world are space-time adjustments, which happen in relation to our surroundings and to other people.

People with Parkinson's have difficulty refining their body awareness, which involves proprioception, as noted above. To move fluidly (easily) through space and time requires people to attune their senses whilst they are moving. This ability to sense ourselves in movement is compromised in Parkinson's. As I pointed out in Chapter 1, for many people with Parkinson's, taking a step can be problematic and beset by freezing, even if they want and intend to move. For someone with Parkinson's the situations described above of the grass, corridor and child often cause episodes of freezing, because Parkinson's disrupts typical rhythms of time and space. Time seems to lengthen through slower thought and movement processes as space condenses; so it becomes more and more difficult to judge how to adapt to even minute changes in the environment.

Dancing provides an embodied experience of space and time. Through dance, a person with Parkinson's can explore the use of time and space consciously. As judgement of space becomes more difficult, so dancing may guide participants to thinking about space and time outside of what Sacks calls the 'Parkinsonian world' ([1973] 1990: 63). Dancing also orientates participants to the conscious execution of tasks and to other people and thus provides a reorientation to the 'real' world. Dancing demands deliberate placing of the body and moving through specific pathways. It has external cues to help participants consciously to execute movement, such as the pulse, mood or imagery of the music, the movement of a dancing partner, or the guidance of the teaching artist.

A popular way to counteract freezing is to put an object in front of the person with Parkinson's, such as a foot or stick, and the person can use this as an external cue in order to step over it and out of the freeze. Because the dancing environment encourages interaction, creative ways of moving and the use of props or other art forms, such as music, it is an ideal place to incorporate tactics to lessen the length of time in a frozen position. One dancer in Bassano del Grappa carries a string of worry beads that he drops in front of him when he gets stuck, or he asks another dancer to stick out his or her leg in front of him so that he can step over it. In a show at B-Motion Festival in Bassano in 2015 in which this dancer performed, sticking a leg out for him to step over became a motif within the choreographic score. A dancer in London asks people to sing *London Bridge is Falling Down* so that she can march herself out of the freeze.

Giving participants the task of improvising a dance creates an environment in which they have a heightened awareness of how their bodies are moving through time and space, possibly more so than in a formal dance class with set sequences to learn. Sacks gives the example of Ed W who goes through an elaborate, improvised sequence of small movements within his body in order to stand up from his chair. Sacks ([1973] 1990) explains that although Ed W's implicit knowledge of how to stand is impaired, each time he gets up, he reinvents explicit pathways in order to do so. Reinventing movement pathways is encouraged in dance improvisations, but even in a didactic dance environment, breaking down a phrase of movement into small sections gives the Parkinson's dancer a road map to navigating the execution of movement. For Sacks this process diverts attention from the transfixed to the conscious so that space begins to expand and time shortens, allowing the conscious activation of movement and tasks to be possible again.

## Exploring qualities of moving

The tactics described in the preceding two paragraphs help normalize the Parkinson's dancer's relationship to space and time. Moreover dance is an aesthetic use of space and time. It is untethered to the usual constraints of functional every day actions. This distinguishes dance from many other physical activities. Movement is conducted in dynamically enhanced or diminished ways, as movement analyst Rudolf Laban theorized in his framework of four 'efforts' (Thornton 1971). Travel through space may be along a direct or indirect pathway. The duration of this travel may be sudden or sustained. The weight contained within the body in its movement trajectory may be light or strong. The flow of movement may be bound or free. The dancer consciously manipulates these 'efforts' or dynamics, intentionally playing with, and colouring, movement states to create qualities in the dancing.

Parkinson's often affects the qualities of movement. Many people particularly affected by bradykinesia and rigidity move in a bound and sustained way (that is, contained and slow), yet often move along indirect pathways and experience a lightness of weight. Others, particularly those affected by dyskinesia, move in a light, indirect pathway, but still with a bound, stuttering sense of flow. The lightweight quality of movement manifests itself, for instance, in a lack of bend in the knees, a hesitation or carefulness, and not striking with the heel when walking, lending movement a floating quality. These habitual patterns of movement are difficult to shift and as a consequence, contribute to the body not being conditioned enough to prevent falls.

Dancing challenges people's dynamic range. Constructing movement patterns, energies, qualities and shapes helps structure how people with Parkinson's may move differently with intention and creativity. In 2010, the English National Ballet's sessions on *Romeo and Juliet* (Nureyev, 1977) used exercises that challenged the participants' habitual qualities of movement. The connection to the emotional intensity of the story helped participants focus on embodying specific movement qualities. For example, normally Mary C moved with a light, delicate quality. Her movement was hesitant and delayed by bradykinesia, and her right arm was sometimes affected by a tremor. Her right arm did not stretch out as much as her left, and her elbows were still bent at the extent of her reach. In dancing Juliet's discovery that her lover (Romeo) had killed her cousin (Tybalt), Mary C made a strong, weighted movement. She leaned forward as instructed and threw her arms out in front, using a strong and powerful dynamic to indicate the anguish Juliet is feeling at that point in the story. The reach in both arms extended through her arms, hands and fingers, now stretching out with a sudden, direct trajectory. Her movement interpretation became so much more alive and vibrant.

Other participants in Mary C's group had a bound flow of movement, made more pronounced by stiffness of muscles and the disjointed quality of uncoordinated movement. The flag dance of the Montague and Capulet entourages required participants to take on more free-flowing, coordinated movement. Participants were asked, through the movement of their arms, to imagine flags or silk curtains fluttering in the breeze. From first using their hands like paws, without articulation, and with a limited flow and range of movement, some participants gradually started to articulate their hands, wrists, elbows and shoulder joints to mimic the rippling of flags. In addition, some began to coordinate both arms to draw figures of eight in the air, or draw symmetrical patterns.

Connected to the ability to convey different dynamic intonations of movement is the ability to communicate the story and the expressive desires of the characters (if only to the participants themselves). Many dance for Parkinson's classes use dancing to create narratives. For English National Ballet, the sessions are often based around stories from ballets in the company's current repertory such as *The Sleeping Beauty* (Petipa, 1890, additions by MacMillan, 1986), *Swan Lake* (Deane, after Petipa and Ivanov, 1997), *Petrushka* (Fokine, 1911) and *Le Jeune Homme et la Mort* (Petit, 1946). Similarly, the Brooklyn Parkinson Group uses stories from dance works performed by the Mark Morris Dance Group. Stories give the opportunity for the abstract colouring of movement to be formed into character-driven exercises. Dancers become a swashbuckling pirate from *Le Corsaire* (Petipa, 1899), heart-broken Dido from *Dido and Aeneas* (Morris, 1989), cheeky Swanhilda from *Coppélia* (Hynd, after Saint-Léon, 1985). The characterization of the movement then becomes easily entwined with telling a story. Other Dance for Parkinson's programmes invent stories around abstract movement in order to help participants remember the steps and to inject a sense of fun. For example, Dance for Health often uses images with which participants are familiar, or are able to imagine – such as picking apples, brushing off the spiders that fall from the tree, stamping on the spiders – in order to let people use movement imaginatively.

Thus, the dancer with Parkinson's can be encouraged to explore what it is like to move in many ways, to carve up new space beyond their habitual spatial zones, to experience moving in time with others. Dancing creates an imaginative, loosely framed opportunity for those with Parkinson's to come out of physically and mentally limiting habitual ways of moving and perceiving.

## With feeling, or the specialness of dance

The chapter has until now concentrated on the objective, material properties of dance and their effects on participants. Dance, however, encourages the dancer (and spectator) to enjoy the feeling that dancing gives him or her. How the experience feels, for good or bad, is one of the primary sensations and lingering after-effects of dance participation and spectatorship. As dance philosopher Anna Pakes states, this experience of sensing how we feel in the moment – this 'phenomenal consciousness' – 'seems crucial to why we value dance, whether we are performing ourselves or watching others perform' (2006: 95). Participants pay most attention to the lived experience when talking about dancing and it is this that allows us to acknowledge the specialness of dance. By referring to the value dancing gives us through how it is experienced subjectively, it is possible to talk about dance as being special.

Some of the early dance for Parkinson's studies recorded statements from participants about how they felt dancing: 'light', 'happier', 'invigorated', 'exhilarated', 'symptom-free' (Westheimer 2008: 8) and 'fun', 'joy', 'pleasure', 'togetherness', 'good' (Heiberger et al. 2011: 8). At the English National Ballet's London class, participants gave similar short answers that characterize their experience: 'exhilarating', 'joyous', 'useful fun', 'satisfying', 'challenging in a positive way', 'magical', 'brilliant' (English National Ballet discussion group 2014a).

The idea of joy as an integral part of the dancing experience is one of Dance for PD's ten key elements of dance that it uses within advocacy, as noted in Chapter 2 (Dance for PD 2011; Bee 2008). Although other feelings may be present, or even more present than joy, joy is a word that continually surfaces in discussion with participants and the use in advocacy makes it a feeling to explore more. As philosopher Brian Massumi asserts, joy is 'affirmation, an assuming by the body of its potentials, its assuming of a posture that intensifies its powers of existence' (2015: 44). Joy allows us to feel totally present in the moment. It is a feeling of belonging to this world and to others, as well as a sense of aliveness. Although it is not the opposite of unhappiness – joy may overwhelm, too – it is an intense feeling that is also 'self-affirming' (Massumi 2015: 45). Both physical and mental, joy imprints a 'desire for life, or for more to life' that calls for us to participate actively together, irrespective of flaws (Massumi 2015). Massumi's definition[7] resonates with Parkinson's dancers' descriptions of joyful feeling and of the value dance has for them, despite infirmity. In Oxford, one dancer explained that after class she feels

> Happy, warm, relaxed and ready for anything but not terribly energetic…. [Warm] means more than one thing. It means happy, content, positive, at one with nature, happy with the world really. You can convince yourself that everything is right.
>
> (Josephine DG 2013)

This statement exudes a sense of contentment; Josephine DG basks in what is sometimes called a 'warm fuzzy glow'. And yet she admits that this feeling is only temporarily transformative. Everything is not right, but the feeling generated from dancing is so positive that she can accept this joyful state.

Jane D'A (2011) from London reports a remark by her carer: 'My carer came today. I told her about English National Ballet. She said, "Pity you can't do it every day. It's good for you, you look different". I was elated and it showed in my face'. Here too, dancing acts as a temporary way of feeling alive that physically and mentally masks the draining effect of Parkinson's. Other descriptions have painted a picture of how invigorating the class can be for people:

> What a buzz there was in the class today. It started quietly, as usual, with breathing and posture, but when it came to movement with words – 'Look at me, not at him' things became very lively. Especially noticeable when one side of the room tried to out-perform the other in gestures and volume. Everyone seemed to forget their infirmities or self-consciousness, and threw themselves whole heartedly into it. When it came to the theatrical marching head up, shoulders back, superior expression, flaunting our own importance! – the change in people went up several notches.
>
> (Jeremy A 2013)

This description vividly captures the energy and conviviality of the dance class. The sense of dynamism created by the participants inventing their own creative path through the exercises is palpable. Sue C describes this process as 're-energizing':

> Sometimes I think I'm so comfy at home that I don't want to make the effort to go out, or I feel miserable and dread going out. But without exception, when I have made the effort to get there I'm *so glad* I did, and being amongst everyone else is a great lift, and I arrive back home feeling really energized. It isn't nearly so much fun doing exercises by oneself. It doesn't re-energize you being on your own.
>
> (Sue C 2013)

It is clear that although these experiences are personal, they are also shared by the group of dancers. The energy of the group carries everyone forward, which to some degree is a testimony to the teaching artist's facilitation of the class.

> The class finished with imagining: we were passing something precious that we had learned from one person to the next. This was extremely touching, everyone really engaged with this and showed great tenderness and care in the exchange. As J. passed it to me she said 'mind it doesn't jump', which quite tickled me.
>
> (Jim S 2013)

The dancers embody the energy physically, vocally and in relation to each other, as well as in the collective imagination of the group.

Jim S' description of an exchange of words and gesture brings out the embodiment of the social connection established through movement and conversation. The dynamic quality of the movement (tender) and the sharing (with care) of each other's imaginative movement are highlighted, as is the sense of fun. As the description above, and the one below, imply, dancing may have a strong emotional core that can be brought out by the connection created between participants.

> Doing ballet [...] is bringing us, the pupils, closer to each other. We have partners for some activities, and for one of them I found myself partnering A, a tall man who I had never seen smile, I think we were both a bit frightened of each other, but after about several minutes working together, we were laughing.
>
> (Josephine DG 2013)

Several Dance for Parkinson's research studies note the social value of dancing. Heiberger and colleagues (2011) found that one of the strongest improvements in terms of quality of life markers was in the quality of people's social life. Hackney and Bennett conclude in their review of quality of life studies linked specifically to Dance for Parkinson's that 'dance is a social activity that could enhance strong supportive relationships between those with PD, their caregivers, and other loved ones' (Hackney and Bennett 2014: 23). Indeed, several participants mentioned that they valued meeting others with the same condition in an environment that made them feel uplifted. Sue C (2013) wrote in her diary: 'One of the chief pleasures of this course has been interacting with other people who have Parkinson's in a happy, easy-going atmosphere where we all have Parkinson's (of varying degrees) in common'. The London Popping for Parkinson's class for people with young onset Parkinson's elicits similar comments. Sarah W (2016) said, 'it [the dancing] has brought us together as a group. It's really nice to see each other every Monday. We've become friends and we've got things we can talk about. We call and say hello. No one else understands'. These comments attest to improved social lives and a feeling of support and communality for each other.

Carers and family members have a similar experience. The daughter of a member of the English National Ballet's Liverpool class wrote in her diary:

> For me, the chance to spend quality time with my Mum and seeing her animated and enjoying the time at the studio are memories I will cherish. We have spent so much time over the past few years at hospitals and clinics. The Parkinson's Dance has given us the chance to share some special time together.
>
> (Sue 2014)

'Special time together' for Sue is not time spent with her mother Betty in medical settings to diagnose and treat her condition, but about time spent enjoying dancing with her. Their dance time underscores the importance of the non-instrumental, of not thinking of dance as a tool to get well, but as dancing as a pleasure for its own sake. For Sue, dancing with Betty is not primarily about addressing her Parkinson's, but about creating a space in which they can interact as mother and daughter.

The connection between Sue and Betty illustrates how dancing not only allows for social interaction, but also for a more intimate way of connecting through movement, which may get lost as adults age. Dancing is a visceral, tactile activity that is displayed through the person, not via a canvas, piano or ceramic pot. There is no intermediary in the execution of aesthetic form and idea. The human body as a vehicle for creating, sensing, relating and communicating is central to dance and dancing. For people with Parkinson's, the opportunity to explore movement in a creative or artistic environment is attractive because it addresses specific challenges and needs, often those of communication and sensation, as well as peaking interest or curiosity. Yet the human body dancing is not merely a tool or instrument. Philosopher Francis Sparshott notes, '[d]ance is peculiar among the fine arts for the way in which it involves the humanity of the artists themselves. Dancers dance with their bodies as instruments, but they dance as people' (1995: 453). Community dancers exemplify this: they dance 'as people' because they may not have a finely tuned 'instrument'. Professional dancers often try to 'disengage' from, and transform, themselves 'as people' through 'non-ordinary' movement (Sparshott 1995: 453), but the community dancer has less physical resources to do this. So their personhood, their humanity, plays an even more distinctive role in the participatory experience and may become a defining quality in any performance or sharing of work that may take place.

Possibly because dancing is intimately connected with the person, participatory dance may connect to individuals on many levels – for example, physical, social, intellectual, emotional, creative, musical, theatrical. So, dancing can be seen as special in different ways, rather than in one particular way. Not all elements are of similar value to Parkinson's dancers, nor to the researchers who study dance for Parkinson's. Moreover, many people with Parkinson's find other activities, such as gardening, cycling, ice skating, tennis and tai chi, beneficial and valuable in several ways. Although dance is special for the reasons described above, this does not mean it is better than these other activities. Some people prefer them to dance. So, although this chapter has established a particular set of valuable characteristics of dancing, its specialness is not necessarily about uniqueness, but about participants valuing the art form because it provides a meaningful experience for them.

Occupational scientists Wilcock and Hocking (2015) lay out criteria for meaningful activity and this may be translated to specific dance for Parkinson's experiences. Dance for Parkinson's initiatives create an environment where positive difference may happen because the dancing event offers four elements: doing, being, belonging and becoming. As an occupation – a regularly occurring, meaningful activity – dancing offers a way for participants to dance (to do), to be a dancer (to be), to belong to the group of dancers and dance organization (to belong) and to realize aspirations irrespective of Parkinson's (to become). Wilcock and Hocking regard these four elements in brackets as crucial to a person's health and well-being.

Context is vital to creating a meaningful experience. For instance, how the sessions are led is fundamental to how they are experienced. Since the experience of participants directly influences the amount of value (or specialness) conferred upon the art form, facilitation becomes an important factor. Leadership in community arts, (arts such as dance, drama or pottery) is characterized by similar principles, as laid out in Chapter 2. They guide the varied ways that teaching artists facilitate work and how they relate to the people who participate in their projects and classes. The mission to make a positive difference, particularly by enabling participants, is the central plank of the practice of many community arts organizations and teaching artists. As one example, Marc Vlemmix from Dance for Health argues that dance for Parkinson's is not special because of the dance, even though he is an advocate for dancing, nor because of Parkinson's, even though he is passionate about ameliorating quality of life for people with Parkinson's. Rather, the key for Dance for Health is facilitating a movement forum away from habitual environments where people may experiment and explore what is possible for them. The focus is on creating an environment that allows participants to take initiative. This, Vlemmix explains, may lead to a participant deciding to change his or her attitude to the disease, or to instigate other changes in his or her life. Vlemmix, who has Parkinson's, is clear that for him, dance for Parkinson's is a lifestyle: he is inspired and empowered by dancing (Vlemmix 2014). Dancing is not just an activity, an exercise class once a week, but a way of living one's life that is inspired by art, rather than by pathology or medical prescription. To illustrate his point, Vlemmix (2014) told me a story. He was sitting in the consulting room and given a long questionnaire to fill in about his Parkinsonian symptoms. The questionnaire would contribute to research on Parkinson's. He gave it back to the consultant unread and told him he was going dancing instead because that made his life meaningful and made him feel good. He had found his way of living well already.

## Notes

1   The priorities were listed as: tackling motor symptoms, which affect balance, falls and fine motor control; non-motor symptoms, especially sleep problems and urinary dysfunction; mental health issues connected with stress, anxiety, dementia and mild cognitive impairments; side effects of medications, including dyskinesia; tackling medical interventions with better monitoring strategies (Deane et al. 2014).

2   Research tasks included the Fullerton Advanced Balance Scale, which had ten movement tasks that the Parkinson's dancers had to complete (Houston and McGill 2013).

3   Rudolf Laban documented these 'planes' to articulate the different spatial areas in which a person can move. Horizontal and vertical perhaps are recognized more readily. The sagittal plane cuts through diagonally between the horizontal and vertical, as in the instance of reaching up to knock on a door.

4   The case for lasting effects of more regular gait pattern is not shared amongst all the studies though. McGill et al. (2018) suggest that gait patterns do not necessarily substantially become more stable after dancing. Using accelerometers to measure gait variability, the study could not find significant differences between the control and experimental groups.

5   These studies specifically looked at fractal dynamics in walking.
6   Dance scholar Valerie Briginshaw (2009) describes the sociocultural marking of space in the dance film *Outside/In* by CandoCo. A kiss is passed along a line of people, female to male, male to male, able bodied to disabled, disabled female to disabled female. The intimacy of the space highlights the normative and transgressive relations between people.
7   Massumi gives credit to Spinoza in following his notion of joy.

**Part 2**

---

The value of dancing with Parkinson's

# Chapter 4

Living well with Parkinson's

L iving well is the theme that reoccurs throughout the rest of the book. This chapter acts as a short introduction to Part 2 in discussing the issues associated with the notion of living well with Parkinson's, as well as reiterating the vital focus on the people who dance. It again underscores the importance of a methodology that examines value and meaning.

The question of how to live well is asked by people who face a degenerative condition. This is true with people living with Parkinson's. It is very easy to slip into negative thoughts, thinking that nothing can be done to improve quality of life. At the time of writing, there is no cure for Parkinson's and searches for a cure are not straightforward.

Despite advances in medicines since the 1960s, such a Parkinson's-free reality is proving elusive. The causes of idiopathic Parkinson's are still uncertain, and until they are proved conclusively, it is doubtful whether scientists will find a cure. The difficulty in finding a cure is compounded by the variety of symptoms, which not everyone presents. It may be possible that Parkinson's comprises actually several conditions, rather than just one (Palfreman 2015). Even if scientists think they may have found a solution, the process of developing and approving medication as safe and effective for patients takes many years.[1]

At the same time, and somewhat contrarily, there is great hope that a cure will be found. For the Parkinson's community, the search for a cure is paramount. In order to find a cure, the cause or causes of the disease need to be found. Hypotheses of the cause of idiopathic Parkinson's range from pesticides (Menegon et al. 1998; Betarbet et al. 2000) to bacteria in the gut (Forsyth et al. 2011; Sheperjans et al. 2015). High-profile charities, such as the Michael J. Fox Foundation, Cure Parkinson's, Parkinson's UK, National Parkinson Foundation and the European Parkinson's Disease Association have fundraised money and regularly plough it into financing scientific studies that might help contribute to the discovery of a cure.[2] The Michael J. Fox Foundation states simply: 'Our single, urgent goal: Eliminate Parkinson's disease in our life time' (Michael J. Fox Foundation 2015). The stress on the urgency of the task clearly signals the understandable impatience of those living with Parkinson's to be free from it.[3]

Many Parkinson's charities invite their members and the general public to help them find a cure, by raising funds for research by taking part in sponsored marathons or cycling tours, for example. Researchers are invited to local Parkinson's groups to talk about the latest advances in scientific study. The dance participants at English National Ballet regularly send me links to the latest research publicity claiming that a cure might be imminent. In my role as a researcher and so, in their eyes, a knowledge-holder, I am asked to respond in

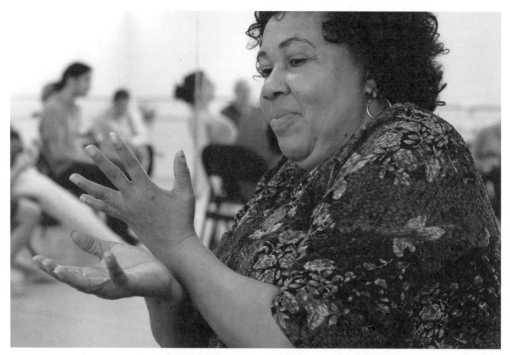

**Figure 4:** Dance for PD at Mark Morris Dance Center, photography by Amber Star Merkens.

helping them divine whether this might be true. The hope that a cure might be imminent is powerful, and many living with Parkinson's are actively seeking to help turn this hope into reality.

The problem of finding a cure leaves those living with Parkinson's with a challenge: how does one live well with a degenerative neurological condition when a cure is not yet forthcoming? The challenge is magnified by the emphasis placed on restitution, on the hope of finding a cure in order to restore people to their pre-Parkinson's state. A restitution narrative accepts that having Parkinson's means a lack and that advances in medical research can fix this lack: 'a person is not whole, not really able, unless one is "cured"' (Stoltzfus and Schumm 2011). Sociologist Arthur Frank (2013) argues that the restitution narrative is seductive in its clean modernist certainty that illness will be converted to wellness, and it is only natural to wish this when taken ill, or after being diagnosed with a neurodegenerative condition. Yet, if healthcare providers and charities have the primary aim of finding a cure, then potentially less emphasis is placed on supporting people to live well with Parkinson's (Goering 2002). Frank notes, '[t]he central problem is how to avoid living a life that is diminished, whether by the disease itself or by others' responses to it' (Frank 2013: xvi).

One challenge to discussing participatory dance's power stems from the dominance of the biomedical model in Parkinson's research. In following a tradition grounded in the belief that things are knowable through empirical testing of cause and effect, most existing Dance for Parkinson's and exercise for Parkinson's research seeks to ascertain the benefit derived from exercise from a clinical point of view: can exercise or dance be proven to alleviate symptoms, aid neuroplasticity, delay disease or even lead to recovery? The research seeks the aspects of dance that most effectively improve functional mobility. Yet, as doctors William Miller and Benjamin Crabtree (2000) argue, knowing the efficacy of a drug (or dance class) is not sufficient to understand how individuals will use it, perceive themselves in relation to it and construct notions of health and illness around it.[4] Yet these uses, perceptions and constructions are important for understanding the user's experience and how the intervention (medication or dance activity) is effective in 'real' life.

Whilst not a cure, dance provides a potent, non-pharmacological response to multiple problems encountered by people with Parkinson's. To study dance's effectiveness and impact outside of medical or scientific paradigms involves investigating the nature of dance and how participants experience it. Questions regarding participants' experience of dancing can lead to discussion of how dance is meaningful for individuals. This may lead to more understanding about why people choose to dance, what it may mean to live well through dancing and what it is about dance in its creative, artistic form that supports therapeutic outcomes. Moreover, investigating dance through examining participants' experience can help scholars explore wider issues concerning construction of identity in the face of a chronic and progressive condition, which has a bearing on studies of ill-being, resilience, disability and social integration.

By way of illustration, over the course of three months in 2013, I regularly visited the English National Ballet class in Oxford. One day, I was waylaid by Sally B, one of the participants, who told me she was being interviewed about the class on local radio later that day. She asked me what she should say. I started to explain that usually the media like to know about how people change physically – in other words, the measurable outcomes – and she stopped me, quite indignant. 'No, no, I don't want to talk about that! It's about how it gets me here', she said as she thumped her chest close to her heart. Sally B's action of thumping her heart communicated that she was finding difficulty in articulating her feelings. Using an action that is understood culturally as symbolic of emotional specialness, passion or intimacy, Sally B indicated the way in which dancing was important to her, which went beyond the physical experience of dancing.

For Sally B, and many others, dancing has a powerful impact because it affects them emotionally, as well as physically or intellectually; it addresses them as individual people, rather than as bodies with disease; it moves them as a group; and it may enrich their lives imaginatively and socially. The role of a researcher is to articulate what all this means and to explain this in order to enhance understanding.

Employing this methodological stance it is possible to explore the reasons why Sally B favours dance because of the way it makes her feel, rather than because it increases her ability to coordinate her arms and legs. Measurement of Sally B's change in mood or energy levels so that she does the housework instead of slumping in her chair will tell us that her mood and energy were altered after dancing, but it will not tell us about the dancing itself, or why Sally chooses to do the housework, or the value of dance for her. A cause-and-effect methodology will not necessarily help us understand the local contexts of dance for Parkinson's, which influence how people access dance, or help us understand people's movement choices and why they feel liberated, challenged, sad or exhilarated. Dance philosopher Anna Pakes notes in her critique of neuroscientific explanations of dance:

> They do seem to leave one crucial dimension out of the picture, namely the lived experience or what it is actually like to perform, create and witness dance. Their focus is on the conditions of experience, not the experience itself. A description of the physiology and neuro-physiology of a dancer raising her arm will not help us appreciate the complex kinaesthetic sensations she feels, or other aspects of her phenomenal experience.
>
> (Pakes 2006: 95)

In concentrating on the measurable, dance for Parkinson's research pushes the non-measurable to a secondary position, despite the questions above being interesting, possibly even important.

The questions relating to the context of action are 'reason-type' questions (McFee 1992). As philosopher Graham McFee (1992) points out, both causal and 'reason-type' explanations play useful roles in our understanding of phenomena such as dance. In fact, he argues that we cannot understand dance without the inclusion of reason-type explanations as well as causal ones. To categorize an event as dance, we cannot resort purely to describing the physical movement because taken out of context, the same physical movement could be used for an entirely different purpose. McFee cites an instance where one could be performing dance-like movement with a broom, but with the goal to sweep up the dust on the floor. He argues that because we cannot rely on categorizing through describing, the context of the action becomes paramount. In examining the context of action, we ask ourselves reason-type questions: 'why' questions, rather than 'what' questions. Both the causal and reason-type explanations are needed because they address different aspects of dancing and can be seen as complementary.

An exploration into people dancing (as opposed to bodies dancing) does not aim to prove something empirically, or to determine causal relationships between variables, but to contribute to greater understanding of the complexity of human existence; of people's perceptions and actions; of the lived experience. The emphasis on people and on the humanity of dancing, rather than on bodies or pathology, offers a way into examining the emotional power and attraction of dance for Parkinson's. Sacks says that, in his work, he felt it important not to forget the person, the subject within the research, rather than concentrating on the disease and its effects. He argues, '[o]ver and above the disorder, and its direct effects, were all the responses of the patients to their sickness. So what confronted one, what one studied, was not just disease or physiology, but *people*, struggling to adapt and survive' (Sacks [1973] 1990: xxviii, original emphasis). He adds:

We have seen Parkinsonians as bodies, but not yet *as beings* […] if we are to achieve any understanding of *what it is like to be Parkinsonian*, of the actual nature of Parkinsonian existence (as opposed to the parameters of Parkinsonian motion), we must adopt a different and complementary approach and language.

(Sacks [1973] 1990: 7, original emphasis)

After reviewing a broad spectrum of literature on the value of cultural activity, arts consultants John Carnwath and Alan Brown go further in stressing the importance of research that focuses on the experiences of arts goers:

It seems fair to say that biometric research is unlikely to provide a practical means of assessing the overall impact or value of cultural experiences, at least not in the near future. While research on the biological functions that underlie the aesthetic experience provides the only truly objective measures of audience responses, it is questionable whether such objective responses – however desirable from a research standpoint – are relevant to the discussion of cultural goods and services. It may be that subjectivity is a defining characteristic of cultural experiences and should therefore be central to the investigation of audience responses.

(Carnwath and Brown 2014: 89)

Participant responses, as well as audience experiences, are also vitally important here in assessing participatory and community arts practices. To obtain a more rounded understanding of participant experiences of dancing and of what dance offers to individuals, the dancers as people need to be part of scholarship in this field (Houston 2011).

The added dimension of understanding the experiences of people dancing, rather than merely the effects of bodies moving, gives the researcher the chance to examine how participating in dancing may contribute to living well with Parkinson's. *Dancing with Parkinson's* takes the view that living well with Parkinson's will mean different things to different people. There is no single definition, nor will dance necessarily be the only means people have of living well. The following chapters contain stories of people who link their dancing with the feeling that their life is enhanced, or enriched by the experience. Parkinson's is a disease that encroaches on people's ability to do things, on their sense of self, slowly clawing their world inwards, diminishing their social sphere, networks and bodily capabilities. The book argues that dancing may enhance rather than diminish and so may be a component of living well with Parkinson's.

The boundaries between disability, illness and wellness are blurred when considering a degenerative condition such as Parkinson's. Many people with Parkinson's do not consider themselves disabled, or ill, and yet many suffer social indignities and barriers to social participation because of their condition. Others articulate the frustration and vulnerability felt when having to deal with unpredictable symptoms that, in their view, rob them of a feeling of wellness or 'normality'. Some are gratified that they feel healthy, even though they have the disease. Many experience all of these feelings and viewpoints at different times in their lives with the condition. Living well with Parkinson's is a constant negotiation between these altering states and feelings. Sociologist Juliet Corbin (2003) argues that in order to feel well with a chronic condition, an individual has to feel capable, that his or her body can carry out tasks adequately, that he or she feels good. Frank (2013) argues that living well is more about how one actively decides to live and share one's understanding of the situation irrespective of whether one feels ill or healthy. Both Corbin and Frank agree that in feeling capable, rather than out of control, a person with a chronic illness is more likely to feel and live well.

In the following chapters I probe the notion of living well with Parkinson's via the stories of dancers. These stories are bound by my own interpretation and analysis of their meaning and importance, thereby giving authority to myself as the outsider, rather than to the dancers with Parkinson's. With this in mind, what the dancers witness and experience may not be adequately expressed by my words,[5] but the themes within the chapters come directly from participants. Here, the participants provided much of the data for producing the analysis and formulating theory.

## Notes

1 See Palfreman (2015) for a historical overview of the many potentially exciting developments that have been dashed after, or even before clinical trials.
2 There are other national Parkinson's charities, such as the Kenyan Africa Parkinson's Disease Foundation, Parkinson's Foundation Uganda and the Indian Parkinson's Disease and Movement Disorder Society, but their main goal is to promote public awareness and help support groups, rather than find a cure.
3 The chapter includes points made in Houston (2011, 2015), namely about restitution and Parkinson's research. These discussions were originally published in *Dance Research Journal*, 47:1, 2015 and in *Dance Research*, 29, 2011 by Edinburgh University Press.
4 Outside of the clinical trial, outcomes from taking medicines are often poorer because people do not necessarily adhere to the strict dosages applied during the trials.
5 See Frank's (2010) discussion on letting stories breathe.

# Chapter 5

Exploring beauty

S ipping tea in Carroll F's flat, we began the interview. Carroll F (2012a), a participant in the English National Ballet's London class, immediately exclaimed: 'The dance class really changed my life. I am much more positive. It's something about the music, rhythm and ballet, which makes you feel lovely. I haven't felt lovely in a long time. This disease is grotesque'.[1]

Carroll F's comment, so passionately articulated, intrigued me. The ramification of her 'feeling lovely' points to a number of issues in thinking about dancing, disability and beauty. In particular, her comment prompts rethinking of the place of beauty within a community dance context and in relation to a chronic degenerative condition. This chapter explores how the participant might ascribe value to dance as art or as a social practice, while dealing with a degenerating and potentially life-changing condition.

I was struck by Carroll F's insistence on the feeling of being beautiful as the most important aspect of participating in the dance class, which did not seem wholly tied to the fact that her movement temporarily becomes more fluid. Carroll F returned to the idea of feeling lovely at the end of the interview, stressing its importance for her:

> I've a feeling these classes are going to be my lifeline. It's a combination of physical exercise, which is superb, but also for me it's a sense of being beautiful again. I feel so degraded with the disease. It's very, very important to me that my body is doing something pretty again […]. This disease is quixotic and dehumanizing. Ballet brings you back to childhood. I just love it; I really, really love it.
>
> (Carroll F 2012a)

Her insistence highlights the gaps in research and evaluation studies, which tend to concentrate on instrumental effects and physical benefit (such as Hackney et al. 2007; Hackney and Earhart 2009, 2010; Volpe et al. 2013). Dance is characterized as a possible means to increase physical aptitude, or to counteract Parkinsonian motor symptoms. These potential outcomes are instrumental in showing measurable clinical benefit to the patient. The idea of feeling lovely does not figure in any assessment. Even the well-used Parkinson's Disease Quality of Life Questionnaire, PDQ-39 (Jenkinson et al. 1997), does not address the topic of beauty. Yet, the dominance of instrumental benefit in Parkinson's research provokes the question as to whether Carroll F's response must be dismissed as irrelevant because feeling lovely in a dance class is inconsequential to the serious business of treating and curing Parkinson's.

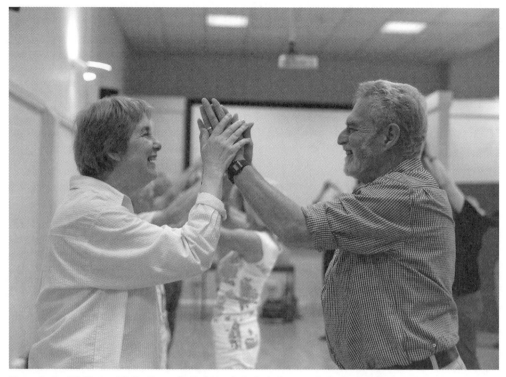

**Figure 5:** English National Ballet Dance for Parkinson's Oxford, photography by Rachel Cherry.

As discussed in Chapter 1, the domain of clinical research into dance for people with Parkinson's is characteristic of a medical conception of Parkinson's and of dance: dance is a means to alleviate symptoms. Indeed, some participants initially are attracted to a dance class because of the possibility (as yet unproven) that it may help slow down the progression of the disease and disablement. This motivation to dance differs from the aims articulated by many dance teaching artists, which as noted in Chapter 2, are focused on participants enjoying dance as an art form and as creative endeavour, rather than as therapy. For example, the teacher training manual for the Dance for PD class explicitly states that the programme 'emphasizes dancing for dancing's sake, rather than focusing on movement as a way to reduce symptoms' and 'emphasizes aesthetic objectives, rather than mechanical, clinical or practical goals' (Dance for PD 2011: 6). Although dancing, not therapy, is the aim, many teaching artists welcome research that indicates symptoms might lessen whilst dancing. Dancing therefore sits at an interesting intellectual and physical intersection between 'alternative therapy' and artistic and social practice.

The previous chapter highlighted the challenge with concentrating on a cure for those who already have Parkinson's who may like to find a way to live well with the condition. Critics of the restitution narrative argue that in pinning all hope and authority on the medical professional or researcher means less space for other ways of addressing the experience of living with a disease that help the person 'reclaim' (Frank 2013: 7) their sense of being a person (rather than a patient) for themselves. The humanity that Carroll F seeks from her position of being 'dehumanized' is her call to reclaim this for herself. Carroll F's call to reclaim her humanity destabilizes the concept that restitution is the only valid narrative for those with Parkinson's.

## The beauty debate

Carroll F's stance on the importance of feeling lovely provokes questions about the status of beauty within dance, in the light of 100 years of philosophical and artistic rebellion against the notion (Danto 2003). The 'disappearance of beauty' (Danto 2003: 6) in twentieth-century modern art and modern dance has created another challenge to discussing beauty as a meaningful concept. Modern art proposed that beauty should not be a necessary condition of art, and so it is less important in discussion of artistic creation. Indeed, Danto notes that 'beautiful' and 'lovely' have become inconsequential exclamations, in the same manner as 'nice': bland and innocuous terms for something pleasing. Philosopher Elaine Scarry describes the situation as a 'conversation' that has been 'banished' (2000: 57), while cultural commentator John Holden observes the 'embarrassment' or contempt conferred upon those who use the term 'beauty' (2004: 23).

Dance scholars within cultural studies and postcolonial traditions have brought to light the dominance of classical ideals of beauty in shaping western aesthetics, as embodied in the principles of classical ballet. Ballet is the dance form that exemplifies the mathematical principles of beauty, where order is produced from the relation between parts. Beauty finds form through line, counterpoise, verticality, symmetry and harmony of elements, as dance critics and teachers have extolled (see Blasis [1820] 1968, for example). Modern dance pioneers and postmodern rebels influenced much of the current philosophical thinking in dance studies. Modern dance not only hit back against the representation of beauty in ballet's disembodied female roles, such as fairies and enchanted swans, but also the manner of their depiction, through disrupting line, harmony and centre of gravity (Wolff 1997). In finding different ways to explore womanhood and other subjects, modern dancers moved away from the classical principles that marked the representation of characters. Many postmodern dance choreographers wanted to explore aesthetic and representational issues that disrupted the classical (and modernist) cannon, as well as sometimes for their work to be situated within a radical political framework (Banes 1987). Because beauty was no longer wanted (or at least, not in the way that was characterized by classicism), it was separated from meaningful sociopolitical engagement, as well as philosophical and critical commentary. Although arguably beauty was still present in many of these choreographers' works, and ballet itself moved on from its classical narratives, beauty in dance is generally seen as apolitical entertainment, nice but inconsequential.

But there is an underlying, more serious issue at play. The dominance of classical principles in, particularly, western thought and art is problematic because the rational way of ordering is formulated as objective and uniform. Because its basis in objectivity is seen as universal and therefore true, classicism has been set up as the tradition offering 'timeless superiority' (Westfall 2010), which means that other forms of expression are seen as subordinate. Postcolonial scholar Bill Ashcroft explains the situation with regard to perspective, a rule-based, classical method of painting, although it translates out to other forms with classical principles:

> The mathematical codification of visual perception is a striking demonstration of the effort to reach a universal viewpoint through the regulation and standardization of individual differences [...]. The discourse of space is one which we enter as we enter ideology. So complete is the success of the perspectival method that this is the way we (Westerners, and increasingly all cultures) understand what the world looks like. And, of course, in one respect it is, but it is not the only, or necessarily most important, way in which the world can be viewed.
>
> (Ashcroft 2001: 136)

It is interesting to note that, as discussed in Chapters 1 and 3, space is one element that is varied and non-standard for those with Parkinson's. Because of this atypical relationship to space, people with Parkinson's often are misunderstood. It is perhaps no accident that Ashcroft argues that perspective creates an 'external fixed position' for the viewer, resulting in the scene soliciting 'no response, no movement towards it on the part of the viewer' (2001: 137). This position creates a problem for empathy, where the viewer sits as an outsider without any encouragement to meet the insider in the scene, to try to understand his or her world and intellectual perspective.

In response, the disability arts movement has done much in recent years to challenge traditional tenets of art, including classical notions of beauty, in order to champion the artistic validity and abilities of disability performers (Garland-Thompson 2002). Carrie Sandahl and Phillip Auslander argue that disabled artists have confronted 'rigid aesthetic conventions' (2005: 4) to break out of the negative and assumed non-creative positions that have been traditionally allocated to them. These oppositions partly derive from the postmodernist rejection of aesthetic theories that propose a universal principle of beauty and thus are exclusionary (Silvers 2002; Eisenhauer 2007). Anita Silvers writes that 'standards of beauty are typically criticized by postmodernists for fortifying patterns of existing power' (Silvers 2002: 229). By 'postmodernists' Silvers means those who 'recognize the personal and political harms that totalizing ideas have visited on people who do not fit into or comply with them' (2002: 228). Like Frank, Silvers acknowledges the need for disabled people to be valued on their own terms.

Disability commentators argue that a universal aesthetic framework excludes people who may not fit the definition of formal beauty. Participation in western concert dance forms is rendered inaccessible to many. Their exclusive technical frameworks reject, for example, those who cannot achieve counterpoise, or who may not produce 'line'[2] (Benjamin 2002). In other words, beauty as a philosophical and political concept has played its part in denying artistic validity to those who subvert that aesthetic because of who they are.

In a similar fashion to the disability rights movement, the community dance movement has espoused the value of inclusive practices, of appreciating an individual's contribution to dancing. Many commentators argue the necessity to move away from external models of 'worth' that impose particular aesthetic presumptions upon community dancers (Lomas 1998; Bartlett 2008). Unlike Sandahl and Auslander's historical portrayal of community arts for disabled people as 'charity' (2005: 1) or 'therapy' (2005: 6), the community dance movement, particularly in the United Kingdom, has sought to champion dancing people as artists, irrespective of how they move or the extent of their formal training. Community dance scholar Christine M. Lomas (1998) argues that this value of dance for all is embedded within teaching methods that acknowledge and celebrate individual ways of moving. Creating dance for and with people with disabilities happens not out of pity, or even for therapy, but because we need to recognize the significance and worth of all individuals and their wish to dance and to create. Critics of the restitution narrative, such as Frank (2013) and Goering (2002), argue for a space where those affected by chronic illness may tell their own stories, away from the technical information proclaimed, prescribed and inscribed onto their bodies by the medical profession. Likewise, disability and community dance scholarship propounds the view that disabled artists (professional and amateur) need to move beyond traditional notions of the beautiful to gain their own powerful, or 'authentic' (Lomas 1998), artistic voice.

The arguments of disability and community dance scholars illustrate the complexity of the notions posed by Carroll F's experience, but do nothing to help understand Carroll F's depth of feeling. Carroll F has a progressive condition that is gradually altering her relationship to movement, space and time, as well as affecting what she is able to do and what she feels she cannot. Exclusion from beauty is apparent to Carroll F in how she conceives of herself in relation to Parkinson's and to her former self, and yet, she invokes beauty – her lifeline and the scourge of many contemporary thinkers – through dancing and participating in a dance class. The primacy of beauty, or loveliness, in Carroll F's experience of dancing calls into question the proposition that beauty has lost its importance within the discourse of community dance and chronic illness.

## A return to beauty

Despite beauty's unpopularity with many theorists, the subject has been undergoing a resurgence since the 1990s (Beckley and Shapiro 1998; Brand 1999, 2000; Banes 2000; Scarry 2000; Eco 2004; Armstrong 2004; Danto 2003; DeFrantz 2005; Winston 2007; Wolff 2006; Thompson 2009). Many of these authors have rejected the old Enlightenment constraints on formal beauty and bypassed postmodern disdain in order to embrace new ideas of what beauty might be. Sociologist Janet Wolff (2006) finds a case to be made for the return to beauty. She and others, such as Elaine Scarry (2000), argue that beauty offers a space for contemplation, reflection and critique. In the words of philosopher Kathleen Higgins, beauty 'encourages a perspective from which our ordinary priorities are up for grabs' (1996: 283). Or, as Scarry poetically puts it, beautiful moments act

> like small tears in the surface of the world that pull us through to some vaster space […] or they lift us […] letting the ground rotate beneath us several inches, so that when we land we find we are standing in a different relation to the world than we were a moment before.
>
> (Scarry 2000: 112)

Linking altered perspective with embodied feeling, Scarry argues that the aesthetics of the beautiful have the potential to generate new lines of thought and new approaches to situations. Once removed from its association with universal aesthetic principles, beauty within its specific artistic, cultural or environmental context can be the basis for talking about fairness and justice (Scarry 2000), social action (DeFrantz 2005), suffering (Thompson 2009) and community values (Wolff 2006). As Wolff points out, social and ideological interests and contexts are implicit in any discussion of the intrinsic value of beautiful art, and these are made explicit within this new 'post-critical' discourse, which not only highlights how people's identities, such as those framed around categories of race, sexuality, gender and ability, are constructed within an artistic context, but also argues within frameworks of value and ethical responsibility. The old critique of beauty as amoral or as an anaesthetic to political action is dismissed. Wolff states, '[m]aking the case for a return to beauty means, among other things, re-thinking the assumption that political art is obliged to disrupt aesthetic pleasure' (2006: 146). And, in light of Carroll F's situation, making the case for the return to beauty means re-thinking the assumption that it may disrupt any serious consideration of identity and affirmation of humanity. As sociologists of art Antoine Hennion and Line Grenier put it:

> The work of re-socialization of art also needs to come closer to art lovers' tastes and practices, without contenting oneself with an external acknowledgment of the value given to art by members of an art world as if art was a belief, and not also an experience of pleasure, expression and emotion collectively lived by subjects and bodies through specific objects and procedures. Asking questions on the political, ethnic and sexual value of art has been a way of showing how art does construct identities, bodies and subjectivities.
>
> (Hennion and Grenier 2000: 341)

The return to beauty for some scholars (DeFrantz 2005; Wolff 2006; Thompson 2009) has involved arguing for a 'principled' beauty (Wolff 2006) that deals with beauty as value, without seeking to universalize: 'Rather than defending absolute or essential moralities and political values, post-critical thought focuses on the emergence and development of shared discourses of value in the context of community [and] inter-community dialogue' (Wolff 2006: 151). Values, such as beauty, are negotiated and developed within a specific context and are seen within the dynamic relationship between thought, action and social structure. Through art, beauty may highlight issues within a shared context in which groups marginalized from traditional discourses of beauty (such as people with Parkinson's) may articulate their aesthetic priorities. Through these discussions, beauty becomes 'a potent and important paradigm for group awareness and well-being' (DeFrantz 2005: 100). As Wolff comments, this 'post-critical' stance is formed through listening to the shared articulations of value within a group that has a 'concept of community' (Wolff 2006: 151). For example, dance studies scholar Thomas DeFrantz (2005) has been able to articulate the value of African American dance through taking into account the social and political interests at the heart of an 'Africanist beauty' and using these as the frame through which to analyse dance works. Performance scholar James Thompson (2009) uses the context of suffering and violence in war-torn communities to demonstrate the value of beauty in participatory theatre as a source of revitalization and hope.

## Experiencing disability

Making sense of Carroll F's passionate affirmation of feeling lovely involves pursuing the value placed on beauty within Carroll F's own situation and as part of a shared understanding within the dance group. In so doing, such an analysis may highlight issues pertinent to the link between aesthetics and health, illness and well-being. At the time of the interview, Carroll F was still in the early stages of disease progression. Despite this, she characterized her condition as 'dehumanizing'. In another aside, she called it 'disgusting and horrible' (Carroll F 2012a). The walls in her sitting room were covered with pictures, including those of her younger, charismatic self as actress, mother and lawyer, and of her late husband in his role as a politician. Dancing between these photographs is the image of beauty, of power and of family life mixed with living in the public eye. Although still active in charity work, Carroll F makes it clear that Parkinson's has created a different feeling about herself and about her body from the image created by the pictures on her wall. As Frank (2013) notes, those who develop chronic illness later in life often find it hard to adjust to living with a life-altering condition.

Moreover, since Parkinson's has a bewildering array of symptoms that occur and change over time, it is often difficult for people to come to terms with the disease because it is not stable. Even if one tries to eliminate social barriers for people with disabilities and even with committed championing of disability rights and achievement, individuals may still struggle personally with an impairment or chronic illness (Swain and French 2000). Disability and performance scholar Petra Kuppers addresses this situation in her two-rooted concept of disability:

> *Disability* is a slippery word that holds nightshade and sunlight, a concept that grows above ground, in our disability culture politics, and below, in the privacy of the disarticulation of pain, of isolation, of the lived reality of social and physical oppression.
>
> (Kuppers 2011: 94)

The affirmative and collective expression of disability has to be understood alongside the individual, often voiceless, expression of hurt. In other words, the manifestation of group positivity may mask an individual's pain and the social obstacles that he or she encounters.

Medical sociologist Michael Bury describes the state of change for people with chronic illness as 'biographical disruption' (Bury 1997: 124), whereby their sense of identity and control over their life is threatened by the onset and progression of disease. Bury identifies two types of concerns, or 'meanings' (Bury 1997: 124), emanating from biographical disruption. The first centres on how symptoms bring a sense of uncertainty to everyday life by interfering with it. As Roy K (2011), one of Carroll F's fellow dancers, notes, 'having Parkinson's makes you insecure because you can't predict what will happen'. In his letter, which features in a European Parkinson's Disease Association (EPDA) support booklet, Skjalvor describes the condition as

> like living with a thief. It controls all my functions, my visual perception, cognition, my mind, blood pressure and body temperature and my sex life. Like a thief in the night, it sneaks up on me and my dignity so that I lose my motor skills and power to control.
>
> (EPDA 2011: 7)

The second concern focuses on the symbolic significance of the disease to the person with the condition. In addition to dealing with specific symptoms, which may have consequences, such as not being able to get dressed by oneself or not being able to write, the person has to deal with the assumptions, prejudice, expectations and roles that social discourse confers upon someone with a named condition. For example, Zofia (2012), another dancer in Carroll F's class, comments that she is 'afraid to be in touch with normal people. I am afraid of being patronized'. John H (2012) notes how he sits on his own at parties, finding it difficult to talk, and Eddie N (2012), at one time a triathlete, speaks of his gradual isolation from his group of sporty friends 'who dropped by the wayside' as his Parkinson's developed. Jorge, another person with Parkinson's whose letter was printed in an EPDA support booklet, writes of his social anxieties brought on by the manifestations of his condition:

> I was invited to an official dinner [...]. The pressure to 'perform' feels too much and the quick 'give-and-take' that is so much part of a normal life is impossible. Parkinson's also makes my voice different and I often speak, involuntarily, in a near whisper. Add to this a face that is empty of expression – the so-called 'Parkinson's Mask' – and you have a clear picture of me as 'a loser' in such situations.
>
> (EPDA 2011: 30)

Isolation, whether self-imposed or involuntary, is a common consequence of the assumption and prejudice of those around people living with the disease. The symbolic significance of the disease is clear in these testimonies of marginalization.

It is in the meanings attached to biographical disruption that beauty meets Parkinson's and where the symbolic significance of beauty is formulated. Carroll F's comments of disgust are typical of many people who have Parkinson's, as is the black humour that colours her conversation. It is interesting to note that scholars and artists have articulated their understanding of disgust by setting it deliberately against beauty (Danto 2003). As with beauty, disgust owes much to morality and social etiquette (Miller 1997). As a moral and social concept, beauty is on a par with goodness and social worth, while disgust signifies a lack of beauty and social value. Self-disgust is linked to embarrassment, a common sufferance for those with Parkinson's, who may isolate themselves socially in order to hide the signs of bodily disorder, or to avoid the reaction of others, as mentioned above. The loss of control over one's body may stand as an embodied symbol of anti-beauty.

A key element of social acceptance is having control over one's actions. As dance studies scholar Ann Cooper Albright notes, the disabled body can be seen as a symbol of the uncontrolled and 'grotesque' (1997: 74), and as a result, disabled people may experience prejudice. In particular, Cooper Albright points out that theatre dance, such as ballet, is associated with hiding pain, sweat and effort, the elements that highlight the struggle with controlling one's body. It is no accident that classical ballet and other dance forms that privilege control are associated with an aesthetic of the beautiful. Dance studies scholar Telroy Davies suggests that to counteract dance's collusion in this cultural phobia of uncontrollability, it is necessary to look anew at movement by dancers with impairments or chronic conditions, seeing it as 'unique, unprecedented and valuable' (2010: 61), and to acknowledge that we all have to 'negotiate with our bodies' in order to perform movement (2010: 61). Davies suggests that this way of thinking allows those with a chronic condition to see themselves as artists.

Bury's concept of biographical disruption may be countered with Davies' argument of reasserting the value of one's own contribution as a dancer with impairment. The loss of control felt at the height of biographical disruption may be approached differently through a re-evaluation of one's life (and life in dance) with disease, where a new, positive identity asserts itself. Thompson examines the link between participatory art, beauty and renewal in his work in war-torn communities. He suggests that seeking out beauty may counteract pain. Local artists that he interviewed in war zones (where violence, pain and disability are commonplace) cried out not for a 'theatre of atrocity' in order to reflect experiences of hurt and hopelessness, 'but for a "theatre of beauty"' (Thompson 2009: 138) in order to awaken possibilities. A theatre of beauty dwells not on the frustrations, isolation, pain and disability many people with Parkinson's experience daily. Instead, a theatre of beauty focuses on participants' abilities, creative explorations and communal endeavours, areas they have not had the chance or the courage to experience since the onset and progression of their condition.

A theatre (or dance) of beauty is 'enlivening rather than depreciating' (Silvers 2002). In dance for people with Parkinson's, the focus is on moving, on creativity, on artistic interpretation and on social interaction, not on disease and disability. With this focus in mind, one may appreciate participants' unique ways of moving without resorting to pity or charity, and participants may value dancing for the shared experience of moving with beauty, not just as exercise. In this way, one may appreciate that Parkinsonian movement expands the notion of what dance can be, just as dance for people with Parkinson's may expand the notion of what beauty can be. Silvers (2002) argues that such an enlivening perspective of art and beauty gives meaning to the diversity of the human condition and, so, I would add, to Parkinson's. Parkinson's is a fact of life for one in 500 people, and as the population ages, this figure is set to rise (Parkinson's UK 2013). Carroll F's experience with dance suggests that even with movement that has many negative consequences and connotations, participants may still reap value in their own abilities.

## Living with Parkinson's

Frank (2013), himself in remission from cancer, argues similarly. He uses the term 'chaos' to describe the periods of panic and powerlessness that can be felt by someone who develops a disability. This chaos is contained through a different way of thinking: thinking about how one *lives* with the condition and connects with others, about how possibility in life can be created. Frank terms this attitude and process of discovery as a quest narrative:

> Time spent being ill ceased to be time taken away from my life. Instead, how I lived with illness became a measure of how well I could craft a life, whether I was ill or healthy. This attitude is the basis of understanding one's story as a quest narrative. Illness remains a nightmare in many ways, but it also becomes a possibility, especially for a more intimate level of connection with others.
>
> (Frank 2013: xv)

Within a quest narrative, dance can become a tool to help craft possibilities.

Some people with Parkinson's have been able to embark on a process of discovery of the potential of their lives as lived with a chronic condition. Robert B joined the English National Ballet class in 2011. He does not use words like 'beautiful' or 'lovely', but his story testifies to the communal power of the dance class and of how it makes him feel good. His journey through Parkinson's and into dance has been a story of a quest to renew his life. Notably, he uses dance to craft meaning in his life. Robert B's quest narrative comes out of a period of chaos. He was in denial that he had Parkinson's for seven years while living in the United States, as he was afraid it would invalidate his health insurance if he admitted to it. His wife left him, taking his business with her. He could not use his car and became house bound, depressed and overweight. Robert B's story concurs with Kuppers' analysis of the disability experience often being 'lonely' (Kuppers 2011: 97).

His quest started when he moved back to London and began dancing. He confesses the dancing 'gave me a little nudge to get on with life […]. It was the dancing, the euphoria, or, I don't know, adrenaline, made me realize there's still life to live for' (Robert B 2013). Echoing Davies' suggestion of valuing his contribution to dancing, Robert B (2013) states: 'I recognize that I lead my life with the cards I'm dealt, rather than wallow in self-pity. It is rewarding for me to see me do what I'm doing'. Although his narrative is different to Carroll F's, he does talk about getting 'that peacock thing' (Robert B 2013), when dressing up for the occasion. When he told me his story, he was wearing a bright lime green jersey, and he noted that he now dresses up for the occasion and gets compliments on how he looks. The social side of the dancing is important for him – he now goes to the theatre, cinema and concerts with a female friend from the group – and he contrasts the 'very solid' camaraderie of the dance group with the way 'people drop you as a friend' when Parkinson's develops (Robert B 2013). He expresses feeling good about himself aesthetically, through what he wears and through dancing, and asserts his quest for changing his life for the better through the company of others, socially and by dancing with them.

Bob Taylor, user involvement advisor for Parkinson's UK, decided to change his life and those of others after his diagnosis of Parkinson's. He wrote a story of his quest for me. In it he becomes evangelical about thinking differently about disease:

> Learning from my own experiences, I feel that the first thing people want to do when they encounter disease is to put a name on it. However what do you do when you have been labeled, deny it, give in to it, or fight it? The situation is not helped by the fact that friends and family often do not know how to deal with it. Often people's perception of anybody with a serious illness or disability is that he or she has lost something, and frequently they do not know how to communicate because of preconceived notions that they are abnormal.
>
> It is my belief that there is another option; embrace it because it is born of me, and to find the answers that lie within me. Every one of us is unique and our illnesses are individual to us. People who lose something, if they are empowered to take the positives from their 'Wake Up' call may realize what gifts they have, & achieve greatness. They no longer want to be 'normal' & moan over what they don't have. Normal means average, routine, standard, ordinary. This is potentially a defining moment in their lives, if they really want to go for it! Their chance to be EXTRAordinary.
>
> (Taylor 2013)

Taylor's words are echoed in Silvers' argument that depictions of disability in art and art created by artists with disabilities affirm the diversity of human biology and history. They offer an expanded vision of beauty, which 'elevates otherness to originality' (Silvers 2002: 241). This affirmation of diversity and originality makes disability meaningful. Silvers gives the example of painter Vincent Van Gogh: 'We apprehend Van Gogh as an original, an amplifier of culture, rather than as a cultural other. So, although disturbing, the extraordinariness of Van Gogh's manner is seen as being meaningful' (2002: 242). She concludes:

Showing that disability is often obscured and undervalued does not suffice to shatter the bonds imposed by routine discourse [...]. We need to shift from repudiating socio-political relations to realigning them by reshaping beauty into a more expansive idea that revitalizes the meaning of disability.

(Silvers 2002: 242)

Although Silvers talks of great artists and Taylor relates everyday stories, their emphases are similar: one may appreciate the diversity of human existence at the same time as valuing the extraordinary within people and art.

An important point to make about the participatory arts context, though, is that it is, on the whole, a group activity. Beauty within a participatory arts context is not about a solitary genius constructing an artful object. The Romantic movement's discourse of the artist as a lone creative talent does not chime with the idea of sharing and participating in making art, regardless of the talent and experience of the artists themselves. In community dance, the focus is on moving with others and sharing the creative enterprise.

Watching Carroll F improvise with fellow dancer Conrad to the music of Stravinsky's *Firebird*, I first see her eyes sparkle as she focuses on her dancing partner. Then she bends to the side, and sustaining the flow of movement, she circles her upper body around to the front and brings her back and head upright. She touches Conrad's elbow, which sharply shifts to the side and his arm unfolds. Lifting his head, he draws a wide arc with his hand in the space to pause above his head. His arm drops gently to touch Carroll F's nose. She laughs. He smiles.

(Houston field notes, English National Ballet London 2012)

The attention here to flow of movement, to its changing qualities, as well as to trajectories in space produces ways of moving that differ from the habitual patterns of everyday actions influenced by Parkinsonian hesitancy, indirection and boundness. What strikes me about Carroll F and Conrad's exchange is not the increased fluidity of movement, although, as noted, this is important, but the engagement and enjoyment between the two dancers that results in a playful dialogue. In this particular context, feeling lovely develops because people come together.

The joyful sharing of beauty through dance, and through talking about the feeling afterwards, bestows communality upon the idea of beauty. A communal experience of beauty is not a universal experience – and those few who felt too overwhelmed by the positive energy of the dance class may testify to this – but it is still a shared experience whose value is conferred by participants. Although beauty in this context is a feeling that individual members of the ballet class have, rather than coming from the gaze of the onlooker, the fact that dancing is a shared experience giving rise to this feeling creates a sense of significance. Robert B's display of feeling lovely is only created for and within the presence of others. Carroll F's experience of feeling lovely is made within the context of group dancing. It is not a question of beauty being objective and universal; it is not. But the fact that feeling lovely arises within a meaningful context shared by others gives it a communal foundation. In Scarry's words, beauty stands 'before the senses' and calls to us (2000: 109). Beauty in this instance draws people together in a generous desire to share and repeat the experience of dance.

Robert B and Carroll F find dancing is a way to re-craft and enrich their lives. Dancing becomes a channel for their journey of discovery and reaffirmation of the self and of others. Through their dance groups, they feel not only good about themselves as individuals (lovely, euphoric, like a peacock), but also a sense of group solidarity. They affirm their humanity with others by seeing their dance companions moving with beauty, as well as more or less fluidly. Their group becomes a vehicle for support in living with their condition, not because it is about Parkinson's but because it is about dancing, validating the ability and creativity of the participants. In the words of Helena L (2014), a class member in Liverpool, it is dance that 'is non-judgemental'. These participants have chosen to take responsibility for their bodies and for what they do with them, despite the loss of motor control. In this way, the dance for Parkinson's initiatives play their part in enacting what Kuppers (2011) calls disability culture. Disability culture is a process that 'can suspend a whole slew of rules, try to undo the history of exclusions that many of its members have experienced when they have heard or felt "you shouldn't be like this"' (Kuppers 2011: 4). Certainly, dance has colluded in exclusions of those with Parkinson's and other movement disorders, as well as older people in general, in many western cultures at least. Indeed, as noted previously, it was only recently that people with Parkinson's were recommended to do any exercise at all. In some quarters, dance has propounded an exclusive beauty aesthetic. Yet Carroll F, Robert B and their companions have seized upon their chance to dance to contradict this aesthetic history and have in the process found the gift of feeling lovely.

Their quest journeys have not ended though, neither has the progression of their Parkinson's. Carroll F and Robert B have found that dancing has opened up new possibilities for them where their condition is at the moment, and for now, dance is helping them experience 'alternative ways of being ill' (Frank 2013: 117). They both feel passionately that dancing is creating a way of being that surmounts biographical disruption and chaos (it is Carroll F's 'lifeline') and nurtures their life beyond passive positions as patients. Feeling lovely is neither a mere nicety nor an irrelevance for those dancing with Parkinson's. Frank acknowledges that 'what is quested for may never be wholly clear, but the quest is defined by the ill person's belief that something is to be gained through the experience' (2013: 115). For the regular attendees of dance for Parkinson's classes, this belief sustains their enthusiasm for moving.

Examining how the concept of beauty is developed and valued within the context of a dance class for people with Parkinson's throws up issues of living with a chronic condition in later life. It enables understanding/exploration of dance's contribution to that life. The context of a dance for Parkinson's class points to a new way of examining beauty that does not ask for a judgement of taste. Nor does it question the veracity of participant comments, but it can emphasize why people may choose to dance despite having movement that has been deemed disordered. In exploring the social contexts in which participants find themselves (or that they create) and in understanding why feeling lovely is important to them, it is clear that dance plays a role in helping individuals feel able and loveable. This experience becomes political because people with Parkinson's often do not feel capable or valued by others, or even by themselves. Dancing is meaningful to Parkinson's dancers because it gives them choice, creativity and responsibility over their bodies. It gives them a sense of freedom in moving and a place where their movement is valued and understood. Feeling lovely can be the result. While beauty may not be measurable in scientific terms, participants' claims to feeling beautiful make it subjectively valid and important to note if dance is to stake its claim as a meaningful social activity. Beauty through dancing becomes more than an incidental aesthetic frippery; it becomes key to formulating a different relationship with their disabling condition. Carroll F's insistence on the importance of feeling lovely points to an artistic activity that helps restructure biographical disruption away from the uncertainty and symbolic significances that Parkinson's brings.

## Notes

1  An earlier version of this chapter appeared in *Dance Research Journal*, 47:1, 2015. It reproduces and extends much of my article.
2  'Line' is a term used by dance teaching artists and dance commentators, particularly those versed in classical ballet. If a dancer has line, she or he is able to produce a classically harmonious line with his or her body, giving the impression that it extends beyond the bounds of the body, out further into the distance. This usually entails using eye line, the neck and tilt of the head, as well as stretching arms and legs, for example, in an arabesque.

# Chapter 6

Interpreting grace

Inclusivity has been a cornerstone of community dance values (People Dancing 2015). Inclusivity means embracing all dances and all dancers, irrespective of whether they struggle to coordinate their bodies or swoop and soar like birds. In contrast, the quality of grace is defined as a particular skill or naturally harmonious relationship between weight, flow and time. Definitions have implied a hierarchy of physical mettle that does not embrace those with clumsiness or disability. Community dance artists purport to welcome individuals to the dance, and celebrate them, regardless of physical or other forms of disability. Because of their democratic intent, community dancers have not promoted grace as an essential value.

This chapter examines grace within dance for participants with Parkinson's. I pose grace not only as an embodied, felt quality, but also as a quality to be witnessed by others. In this chapter I reassess the aesthetic value of grace and in doing so I argue for it to be articulated through three notions: flow, dignity and gift, adapting the concepts for a secular, dance-based context.

Historically, the concept of grace has inhabited different bodies to those with Parkinson's. It has carried assumptions that are not kind to the mover with Parkinson's. Indeed, Parkinsonian movement can be seen as the antithesis of traditional notions of grace in its tendency towards jerkiness, clumsiness and irregular, small movements. Yet dancers with Parkinson's often talk about feeling graceful while dancing; for instance, Pat C and Jane D'A from the English National Ballet London class:

Pat C: 'I'd say I feel graceful'.

Jane D'A: 'Yes, graceful and elegant, you do [feel that] when moving that way. So often we do actions clumsily and now you aren't clumsy any more when dancing'.

(Pat C and Jane D'A 2013)

The journalist and filmmaker Dave Iverson publicly connected Parkinson's dancers to grace in 2014. Iverson, who has the condition himself, named his award-winning documentary on the Brooklyn Parkinson Group, *Capturing Grace*.[1] Dancers with Parkinson's suggest that grace might be a significant aesthetic quality to them and so in this chapter I aim to articulate the ways in which grace might be present in their dancing lives.

I explore what grace can mean, historically, as well as specifically to those with Parkinson's, weaving historical and theoretical ideas of grace together with the context of dancing with Parkinson's. I take three explorations of grace to re-characterize this aesthetic quality for

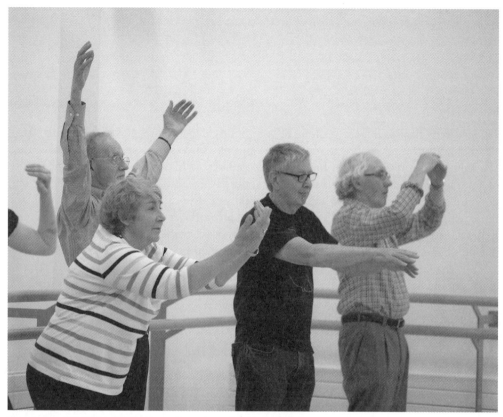

**Figure 6:** English National Ballet Dance for Parkinson's Ipswich, photography by Rachel Cherry.

people with Parkinson's: physical grace, dignity and grace as gift. Through these, the chapter discusses Parkinson's dancers' affinity with grace and the constitutive elements that might comprise the aesthetic quality for people with a movement disorder.

## What is grace?

Grace as a concept has been expounded upon since ancient Greek and Roman times, but came to the fore in art theory during the Renaissance and in philosophical aesthetics during the Enlightenment. Early essays by Dionysius of Halicarnassus, Pliny the Elder, Cicero and Quintilian strongly influenced writers and artists from the fifteenth century onward (Monk 1944) so that grace entered the western canon of art history and philosophy of art as a desirable attribute. Paradoxically, writers did not attempt a precise definition of grace, maintaining that it could not be analysed. In their view, it was not connected to reason, but instead embodied a pleasing, yet elusive quality, a certain *je ne sais quoi* (Monk 1944). Giorgio Vasari ([1550] 1991), the sixteenth-century art theorist, maintained that while beauty was rule-bound, grace was not. Several writers allied grace to a naturalness that would then be 'worked up' by artists of genius (Monk 1944).

Two umbrella concepts were commonly ascribed to grace, which stood for a cluster of descriptive words associated with the notion: *venustas* (charm, loveliness, beauty) and *gratia* (kindness, favour, gratification). Discussion of these deemed that grace in the service of art was achieved by an effortlessness, where the artist departed from the strict adherence to the rules of the art form, be it dance, painting or rhetoric, and brought to it 'a certaine kind of negligent diligence' (Junius cited in Monk 1944: 144). The naturalism of the graceful action was evident in the idea of movement that looks uncontrived, or is carried out with a kind of off-handedness. In writing about dance at the Italian court in the sixteenth century, Castiglione described grace as *sprezzatura*, 'a certain nonchalance' (Castiglione cited in Nevile 1991: 4), that is, without affectation. Writers acknowledged, though, that this ease is an admirable skill and only accomplished through diligence.

Grace has been allied with dancing since ancient Greek times, particularly in the form of the Three Graces, who first appeared in Homer's *Iliad* and became a recurring subject in European art in the fifteenth to eighteenth centuries. From Botticelli's *Primavera* (ca. 1482) to Edmund Spencer's *Faerie Queene* (1590) to Antonio Canova's statue *The Three Graces* (1817), grace has been embodied in art through the figures of three women, often depicted dancing. Opinions differ about what they represent in each artwork: artistic skills, such as dancing, music and rhetoric; or qualities, such as elegance, harmony and charity (Snare 1971); or brightness, joy and gladness (Cohen 1982). The trio is often shown with the goddess of love, Venus, who shares some of their qualities (Gombrich 1945), but the precise nature of her relationship to them is uncertain. Dance scholar Selma Jeanne Cohen (1982) argues that, in the myth of the Judgement of Paris, Venus brings grace into being through an enticing, languid, delicately sensuous dance.

In the sixteenth century, grace was aligned with moral discourse. For example, in describing the rise and fall of the dancer's steps, Castiglione drew upon the commonly held link between graceful dancing and moral goodness. The opening up of the moving body to heaven in the rise reflected the relationship of a person's soul to the cosmos: graceful movement meant a purer soul. The type of movement seen as graceful, characterized by a smooth rise and fall, was only practised by courtiers and royalty, however; so grace entered a social hierarchy where the privileged were represented as being the most moral (Nevile 1991). Thus, grace has the aura of elitism, and this carries through to the dance form that evolved from court dances, ballet. Moreover, the aesthetic of ballet arguably is associated most closely with grace.

In a different way, Modernist writers, such as evolutionary philosopher Herbert Spencer, also privileged the graceful as the most desirable movement quality. In keeping with the industrial spirit of nineteenth-century capitalism, Spencer termed grace as an 'economy of effort' (1891: 383). Ease, he maintained, is brought about through efficiency of movement characterized by an unfussy clarity of momentum that prevents the body fatiguing quickly. Spencer's discourse of efficiency, so relevant to industrialization, can be seen as privileging disciplined, efficient bodies and movement. He disparagingly states:

> No one praises as graceful, a walk that is irregular or jerking, and so displays a waste of power. No one sees any beauty in the waddle of a fat man, or the trembling limbs of an invalid, in both of which effort is made visible
>
> (Spencer 1891: 382)

Spencer's descriptions could apply to those with Parkinson's. In addition to comments on the 'trembling invalid' and 'irregular' stride (Spencer 1891: 382), Spencer tellingly talks of fatigue, which often is felt by those with Parkinson's after moving in a way that expends energy. Although Spencer does not explicitly talk about Parkinson's, his discussion below of those who do not use the 'proper disposal of the arms' sounds familiar and highlights Spencer's impression that walking without ease creates challenges:

> Those who fail in overcoming this difficulty give the spectator the impression that their arms are a trouble to them; they are held stiffly in some meaningless attitude, at an obvious expense of power; they are checked from swinging in the directions in which they would naturally swing; or they are so moved that, instead of helping to maintain equilibrium, they endanger it.
>
> (Spencer 1891: 382)

The parallel between Spencer's description and the asymmetric walk of many with Parkinson's, where the arms do not swing in opposition to the legs, is striking.

Spencer attributes the momentum that he sees within graceful movement as 'curved' motion, a 'continuity, flowingness' (1891: 384) of the body or of a movement, as opposed to the stop-start motion of broken up, 'straight' movement, which punctuates specific points in time. The graceful dancer, creating a sense of seamless action, controls the flow from one movement to the next. Philosopher Henri Bergson writes: 'If curves are more graceful than broken lines, the reason is that, while a curved line changes its direction at every moment, every new direction is indicated in the preceding one' (1910: 12). The trace of ease of the previous movement is felt in the present movement; the trajectory of a past movement can be seen in a present one, as can the intention of a future movement. For the spectator, therefore, the overall effect of graceful movement is the illusion of suspending time, of putting time on hold, because the sense of flow keeps the movement extending (Levin 1983). There is a sense of condensing past, present and future time (Manning 2009). Dance scholar Sondra Horton Fraleigh talks of grace as 'mastering the flow of time' (1987: 99). If graceful movement is bound up in control over the body's temporal mechanics, then those with Parkinson's are condemned to lack grace, sentenced to be chained to the body's functions – to a body that may move in a stop-start fashion, whose quality of movement is bound and weighted[2] by rigid muscles and whose trajectory of movement is a straight line (unless it possesses uncontrolled dyskinesia).

But when dancing, those with Parkinson's talk of a different way of moving and feeling to that described by Spencer and others. For Pat C and Jane D'A, grace is bound up with *feelings* of beauty and elegance. The feelings are pleasurable and very real for them. Their experience points to a more complex scenario, as hinted at by Iverson (2014a), where grace not only plays a part physically, but also in other, more emotionally charged ways. In order to conceive of grace as being part of the dancing experience for a person with Parkinson's, I maintain that it is important to counteract the moral hierarchy, as propounded by theorists of grace. In doing so, it is possible to reconfigure the notions of dancing grace for community dancers with a neurodegenerative condition.

No theories of how community dancers achieve and experience grace exist; this is the first. The literature focuses on the experienced dancer. As noted above, a recurrent theme in writings on grace is the idea of effortless movement and a sense of flow, achieved by great skill on the part of the artist, as well as natural talent, according to some. Theorists in the Renaissance held up as examples artists who had years of training and thus accumulated a thorough understanding of their art form. Castiglione, for instance, stresses the practice and training required to perfect the rise and fall of the court dances (Nevile 1991). No theorists, however, considered how people without much training in dance might achieve gracefulness, unless they were 'naturally' graceful. In addition, most writers concentrate on the artist's relationship with the spectators and their reaction to witnessing grace. Few comment on what gracefulness feels like from the dancer's point of view, apart from speculation that it is a pleasurable sensation. The discussion below sets out my approach to, and theoretical ideas on, grace in relation to the community dancer living with Parkinson's.

## Physical grace

Grace is not amongst the terms chosen to describe the walking pattern of a person with Parkinson's. The gait of people with Parkinson's is often classified as stilted and uncoordinated. The struggle to attain grace as defined above is real. Yet, as Jane D'A explained, dancing appears to help many feel less clumsy. This is backed up by scientific evidence. Factors of movement efficiency and balance have been correlated with the capacity to develop or maintain physical fluency. Studies measuring the quickness of movement, as well as ability to stabilize in people with Parkinson's before and after class also suggest some shift in the way the dancers walk and balance. In an influential controlled study of the effects of Argentine tango and a group exercise class on people with Parkinson's, Hackney et al. (2007) found that only the tango group showed improvement across all the measures of balance and gait, and demonstrated fewer falls. The authors reason that this is because tango is composed of steps that promote dynamic stability, or the ability to return to balance during a dance phrase that takes the dancer off-balance. Argentine tango is largely improvised, the 'leader' in the couple – the dancer who is tasked with deciding what to do – may choose to move in any direction using any step and is free to interpret the rhythms and tempo of the music, requiring the 'follower' to remain hovering in dynamic stillness, waiting for the moment to respond. Dynamic stability – the skill to stabilize during moments of being off-balance – allows for quick changes of direction and weight that give more fluency, less stiltedness. Within this improvisatory environment of tango, dancers play with instability, challenging the ability of the body to remain on balance.

Hackney, Kantorovich and Earhart's findings are interesting when set against Carlo Blasis' discussion of grace as being the dynamic tipping point from balance to off-balance, from stability to chaos. Blasis, ballet master and author of an influential dance manual of 1828, realized that technical execution of movement was linked to the poetics of dancing and thereby to grace (Brandstetter 2005). Unlike the philosophers cited above, Blasis describes grace in terms of physics. He argues that it resides in the moment, for example, when the ballet dancer is performing an arabesque, calling on knowledge of counterbalance in order to stay in a position of equilibrium. The dancer's centre of gravity is so high and the energy greatest when the dancer reaches the maximum stretch on the arabesque that the dancer could easily lose balance. This skill of mastering the vertiginous forces of movement gives the dancer grace. In another example highlighted by dance scholar Gabriele Brandstetter, Blasis identifies the pirouette as a step that can potentially move into chaos because the dynamism and force of the movement may cause the dancer to fall 'out of the "line of gravity"' (Brandstetter 2005: 74) if she or he loses control. As Erin Manning proposes, grace is 'the feeling of being in the eye of the storm, where calm reigns' (2009: 97). This mastery, always on the edge of chaos, gives the spectator the pleasure of seeing grace and the dancer the thrill of moving with grace. Even on the level of a simple movement, such as a grand battement (a swishing kick of one leg), Blasis' idea is useful in describing the tension between stability and instability and the thrill of feeling graceful through the pull between chaos and order.

Contact improvisation is a practice that plays with weight, gravity, momentum and inertia, and lies between chaos and order. Dancers remain in contact with each other to sense moments that may offer the possibility of moving, moments of weight change, pressure of touch, momentum and so on. In contact improvisation, the dancers play with dynamic stability and gravity through giving their weight to their partner and receiving their partner's weight in return, conversing through the pressure of their bodies in unplanned movement situations. It relies on being sensitively aware of the other person in movement and stillness and a readiness to move in response to this awareness in order to build momentum and fluidity. In a 2010 study, contact improvisers with Parkinson's were measured in terms of changes in their ability to walk and balance (Marchant et al. 2010). Although the measurements did not capitalize on the main elements of contact improvisation, the study did indicate an improvement in skills, such as balance and walking, which would be trained by practising transference of weight and changes of direction, weight and velocity. Their balance improved, and the amount of time they spent in the swing phase of the walk increased after ten sessions over a period of two weeks. The study suggests that the participants gained skill in their ability to take and give weight and thus to play with the dynamic exchange between stability (being centred in order to support weight) and off-balance (giving into gravity while being taken off-axis). When this exchange of weight 'works' in contact improvisation, a conversational flow is created between the dancing partners. Fraleigh describes the practice of contact improvisation as 'a spontaneous play of energies as they [the dancers] easily (but sometimes with amazing speed) lift, catch, support, and bounce off each other' (1987: 101). There are echoes of a Renaissance notion of graceful movement here, where easiness of movement is paired with agility. Fraleigh surmises that 'when it works, a magical grace is created, which grows out of an open center' (1987: 101). The openness that Fraleigh describes is the easy bodily state that improvisers develop in order to help them within the improvisatory setting. To negotiate the predictable and unpredictable changes between stability and instability, the body needs to be relaxed enough to be able to alter its direction or absorb the force of another body or object. This is done with a sense of momentum and flow to keep the movement going.

The movement techniques described above may afford the participant dancer tools to develop more physical fluidity. Improvisational dance challenges and encourages a person's capacity to invent in the moment. Improvisation produces movement without copying a teaching artist and ways of moving can emerge that are different to the dancer's habitual style. At the same time, these new approaches to movement can often increase movement flow in a dancer. In the Störung/Hafraah initiative in Freiburg, Germany (2014–15), dance artists, postgraduate scientists and people with Parkinson's worked together to explore this proposition as part of a larger discussion about how dancing might stimulate thinking about movement within the context of movement disorder. The initiative was an international research project with neuroscientists, people with Parkinson's and choreographers. They reflected together on the outcomes of deliberately stepping away from their own movement and conceptual habits and methodologies. Monica Gillette, lead dance artist on the Störung/Hafraah initiative, describes a movement task undertaken by both people with Parkinson's and the postgraduate scholars:

A couple of months ago, the choreographers Matan Zamir and Nicola Mascia were in Freiburg for their residency time and through participating in their classes, I understood a new outcome of what I have identified as physical thinking: When the Parkinson's dancers were given sophisticated movement tasks (on the professional dance level) as opposed to forms to follow, their own bodies guided them into new possibilities. By trying to answer physical propositions, there was space and guidance for their own bodies to physically think towards a solution and often they were able to move like they never had before because they were responding to the movement proposals with their bodies on a physical search. They were not trying to accomplish certain tasks or forms, but rather they were in a process of questioning what is possible through their own bodies. They were seemingly far away from the limitations of their bodies and very focused on following the movement proposals. Their bodies led the way to new physical abilities.

(Gillette 2015)

Gillette identifies that using one's own body to think through physical pathways may often lead to more movement possibilities and, consequently, increased flow of movement than learning a suggested routine, or embodying a specific dance form. Each person has a unique advantage in sensing how to push and develop their own ways of moving. Chapter 8 relates in more detail one of Zamir and Mascia's movement tasks where dancers with Parkinson's take up a series of movement suggestions. They explore space from the floor, as well as standing; they weave in and out of shapes others make; they stand on one leg; they move together. They become more confident with their movement abilities. Further to this, movement softens and limbs lengthen, dancers deliberately put themselves in an off-balance position and carry the momentum from that state of falling into a place of control again. Risk gives energy, and relaxed control gives fluidity. The play between these states manifests itself in how the Parkinson's dancers and others attempt the task. The awareness of possibility brought about by questioning habitual movement patterns expands the pathways discovered and allows the performer to sense in the moment a feeling of gracefulness.

Dancing enables amateur dancers to become more aware of their own and their companion's moving body. The heightened sensitivity to how they and their partners are moving helps deepen and quicken communication and thus eases movement. In addition, ideas to aid the improvisation of movement help deepen physical alertness. Perhaps the examples above of the changed movement of Parkinson's dancers could not yet be termed graceful to an outside eye, but I argue that the shift to moving more easily, with more fluidity, is so marked that community dancers realize something momentous is happening, which, because they are dancing, they call gracefulness. Dance philosopher Francis Sparshott points out:

We must remind ourselves that what immediately confronts us is not a mysterious reality of which 'grace' is the name, but the endless multiplicity of occasions when people use the word 'grace' to apply to things of their own choosing, in situations and for reasons that reflect the histories and strategies of their own lives as they are living them at that moment.

(Sparshott 1995: 334)

In other words, the use of grace when dancing is context specific, special and may be used by those who are community dancers. Cyndy, in the film *Capturing Grace* describes her feeling of grace as having a particular effect on her body: 'My feet feel like glue on the floor. I can't walk but I can dance. The music can lead me, take me to some other place where you're weightless and your body just flies' (Iverson 2014a). The weightless effect that she feels is in relation to her Parkinson's and although weightlessness is part of the discourse on grace (Levin 1983), we cannot understand the full extent and force of her comment unless we also know the Parkinsonian context.

## Witnessing grace

The change in physical gracefulness is not kept as an internal feeling. Others witness it. Grace is a shifting dynamic force owned and recognized by the person who witnesses it and the person who feels it. Witnessing implies that physical grace is wrapped up in the cognitive, emotive and social. Those dancing with Parkinson's certainly recognize that grace is present in their classes, even if they only witness it in someone else. (For example, Jim S wrote in his diary: 'Danielle and the other girl [class teachers] [...] are so graceful in every little movement – there is nothing random; every move seems to have purpose and poise. When I pick my leg up, my foot simply hangs off the bottom' [Jim S 2013]). Witnesses most often comment on the change in physical ability in those who are perceived as being the most disabled. Writing in his diary, Jeremy A from the English National Ballet's Oxford class commented on witnessing arguably the most disabled person in the group march across the floor:

> C, who had started back at the 'taster' session in a wheelchair and was helped out for a brief while, also managed a 'stride' across the room. Initially he had started by shuffling, but in his final turn he managed to put one foot in front of the other, with his helper walking alongside with just a hand under one elbow to keep him steady. We were nearly all in tears. It was very moving – almost like a miracle.
>
> (Jeremy A 2013)

The mystery evoked in Jeremy A's phrase 'almost like a miracle' fits with the language used by Renaissance writers, where grace is seen as unfathomable, unable to be analysed. But however mysterious or compulsive grace might seem to participants, the signs of increased fluidity are noticeable. Sally B (in discussion group 2013b) observed in C: 'What's really stuck me during the last two weeks is the fluidity. The real one is C. Last week he walked unattended. This week his strides were so big'.

These statements (and those in the literature on grace) support the notion that witnessing physical grace implies more than noticing. Rather, there is a sense of connection between the dancer and the observer. For those watching C, there is a sense of witnessing a special act that has a particular meaning and poignancy for those watching. C does not normally move like this, and now he is. The witnesses also move like C, or feel that they will do in a few years, and they understand the enormity of what they are witnessing. Historical accounts also mention the connection to the viewer that a mover might inspire. Spencer (1891) and Bergson (1910) were particularly interested in what they understood as the spectator's sympathy with a graceful mover. Spencer ventures that in the presence of grace, the spectator experiences the same pleasure felt by the graceful mover, and a vague frisson in his or her own muscles, as if dancing:

> When their motions are violent or awkward, we feel in a slight degree the disagreeable sensations which we should have if they were our own. When they are easy, we sympathise with the pleasant sensations they imply in those exhibiting them.
>
> (Spencer 1891: 386)

Bergson suggests that the sympathy the watcher feels is bound up in how he or she senses the fluid rhythm of the movement in his or her own body so that there is an embodied connection with the graceful dancer.

These nineteenth- and early twentieth-century theories of embodied sympathy are precursors to cognitive neuroscience substantive proposals of 'kinesthetic empathy' in the late twentieth and early twenty-first century, which allege that our mirror neuron system causes our muscles to twitch in response to movement we see. Within discussion of kinesthetic empathy a link to grace and ease of movement is implied, noted or claimed (Montero 2016; Foster 2011). The idea of kinesthetic empathy, as it pertains to the mirror neuron system,[3] is derived from experiments that show activity in parietal-pre-motor circuits when we are executing a movement and also the same, or similar, activity when we observe someone else doing the same movement. Proponents argue that the results of studies on macaques (Rizzolatti et al. 1996; Gallese and Goldman 1998) suggest that when watching familiar movement, we are not just passive observers, but enact (or mirror) the actions in our brains. In other words, we register the movement not only on a visual level, but if the movement is familiar, also cognitively at a motor level (Calvo-Merino et al. 2005, 2006). Moreover, two studies examining professional dancers (Calvo-Merino et al. 2005, 2006) found that they had an increased propensity for brain activity when watching a dance movement than the non-trained controls did. In addition to the conclusion that 'the "mirror system" integrates observed actions of others with an individual's personal motor repertoire' (Calvo-Merino 2005: 1243), the results may suggest that physical training in dance heightens perception of dance movement (Davies 2013; Calvo-Merino et al. 2005, 2006), and even proprioception (Montero 2006, 2016). As reported in Chapter 3, proprioception, the awareness of one's own body in space, often is impaired in people with Parkinson's, but there is an argument to be made, helped by Calvo-Merino's experiments, that regular dancing might sharpen proprioception. Better proprioception may lead to more coordinated and controlled movement.

Whether or not these studies help us understand more about grace is opaque, but in response, philosopher of the mind Barbara Montero (2016) suggests that heightened proprioception increases our ability to judge what is graceful in ourselves and others. She states: 'I argue that via proprioception dancers have a conscious, conceptualized experience of the aesthetic properties of their own movements: an experience of their movements as beautiful, or graceful, or powerful, and so forth' (Montero 2016: 193). Montero goes on:

I take my own bodily movements to be proprioceptively graceful, in part because I judge that if seen, these movements would look graceful, and I take certain bodily movements of others to be *visually* graceful, in part because I judge that if I were to move in this way, these movements would feel graceful.

(Montero 2016: 207, original emphasis)

The theory of kinesthetic empathy does raise the interesting idea that those with movement deficit may have the capacity to watch once-familiar movement and recognize it in the part of the brain that deals with movement. This capacity may come alive when in the company of professional dancers who move with ease and fluidity, as is the case in many of the dance for Parkinson's programmes, which use professional dancers to teach, or to assist with the classes. English National Ballet provides a good example where the dance teaching artists and several of the assistants have been through dance training, and for some like Rebecca Trevitt ('Becky') have been, or still are, professional dancers. Carroll F commented to a television journalist:

One of the ballet teachers, Becky, she's very, very special and I watch her during the class and imitate her. And for brief moments of time I can make myself believe that I can really look and move like she's moving.

(Channel 4 News 2015)

In other words, when watching a performer dance, mirror neurons may make us feel as if we are dancing with the same ease and fluidity. If the second conclusion resulting from experiments by Calvo-Merino and colleagues is correct, then perception of aesthetic qualities of movement, such as grace, may be part of this cognition.[4] These conclusions hint at one of the mechanisms for the intimate connection that dancing together and witnessing others dance may bring about: sensing each other empathetically (Foster 2011; Batson 2014).

The work on the human mirror system is in its infancy, with much still to investigate in terms of its relation to qualities and experience of movement. The conclusions outlined here have their critics (Conroy 2013; Davies 2013, 2014). The existence of mirror neurons in humans and, if they do exist, their relationship to learning and control mechanisms are contested. See philosopher David Davies (2013) for a useful summary of the counter-arguments. Glenna Batson (2014) and Maxine Sheets-Johnstone (1999, 2011) point out that movement is constituted of much more than neuronal firings, and so needs to be examined more broadly in terms of its philosophical, social and epistemological implications. Moreover, in exploring empathy within movement, dance scholar Susan Leigh Foster (2011) argues that it is perceived and experienced in culturally and individually diverse ways and so it is important also to acknowledge the specificity of the connections, rather than assuming its biological universalism. Yet, physical grace, which as a concept encompasses the cognitive, emotional and social, could be a springboard to recognizing grace's wider importance, particularly in a community dance context. In creating a feeling of physical grace within both dancer and witness – a shared connection – the concept of 'we' appears. The phenomenologist Edith Stein elaborated on this idea in 1917, which Foster summarizes:

> For Stein empathy was the bodily experience of feeling connected to the other, while at the same time knowing that one was not experiencing directly the other's movements or feelings [...]. Rather than a feeling of oneness with others, empathy affirmed difference and connectedness, offering the means of enriching one's own experience.
>
> (Foster 2011: 164)

In a community context, the concept of kinesthetic empathy as 'we' is seen within the group environment, where people move in diverse ways, yet feel a sense of connection to others in the room, as seen in the case of witnessing C move. *Capturing Grace* director Dave Iverson describes grace in the context of dancing with Parkinson's as a rediscovery that is a communal experience, which goes further in fulfilling each person:

> This is a film about rediscovery, the rediscovery of a lighter step and the sweetness of motion. And it's a story about a remarkable community of dancers – some professional, some not – but all coming together to move in space and in doing so, rediscovering grace. And it is in that rediscovery that each becomes whole.
>
> (Iverson 2014b)

Iverson's statement implies that it is only through moving together that this happens. I contend that the empathetic 'we' is there in the grace of the lightness and sweetness of the Parkinson's dancers' movement.

I suggest in the next two sections of this chapter why this sense of connection may enrich the experience of the community dancer through two characterizations of grace that speak to that experience and which expand the concept of physical grace through the notion of connectedness. These characterizations are dignity and gift.

## Grace as dignity

Dignity is encapsulated in the physical and verbal respect given by someone to another, where the receiver's choices are acknowledged and voice is heard. It is captured in the composed receipt of the attentions of another (respectful or not). It resides in the care and compassion that is shown to a person, so that his or her worth and value as a human being is upheld. Dignity is imprinted on bodies and in actions, as well as in the relation between different bodies and their actions. It helps release the capability of a person through the respectful and care-filled actions of another. Dignity is the empathetic 'we' of physical grace.

At Mark Morris Dance Center, Sharon Resen, a participant, recognizes that witnessing grace in others is as important as recognizing it in oneself:

> I feel graceful, which you don't normally do when you have Parkinson's. You're very often clumsy. You walk in a clumsy way and you feel uncomfortable about the way you look or the way others perceive you. And when you're in that class you feel totally graceful. I look around and everyone else is beautiful and graceful too and it's such a warm and wonderful feeling.

> (Resen cited in Spink and Kim n.d.)

Sharon's perceptions are similar to Pat C and Jane D'A's cited at the beginning of the chapter – grace becomes part of a valued sense of self and of a valued interaction with others. Here is the dignity that dance offers to these participants, a composure that is not always forthcoming in everyday life. Furthermore, respecting others in their dancing confers a sense of dignity on those others also. The idea of dignity is crucial to understanding grace further.

As noted in Chapter 5, lack of dignity is often related to people's experiences of Parkinson's. Some dance participants describe humiliating experiences of being assumed drunk or simple minded. One man got thrown out of a department store for seeming drunk. He was just having a dyskinetic moment, common for those with Parkinson's. Others have felt cause to hide shaking limbs in public, feeling embarrassed by the atypical movement. One dancer related that two young men started filming him with their phones and calling out cruel names because he was walking in a non-normative fashion. Sociologists working in the field of Parkinson's point out that shame is one of its by-products and an emotional reaction to feeling undignified. In listening to the life stories of people with Parkinson's, Gerhard Nijhof (1995) found that the concept of shame occurs regularly in their narratives. He records the indications of the emotion surfacing in his interviews:

> The direct use of the word itself; words considered as its equivalent, such as 'embarrassed', 'awkward' and 'disgrace'; words like 'terrible' and 'horribly' when used with disqualifying connotations; indirect references such as speaking of efforts 'to hide' signs of the disease or of 'not daring something' because of the recognition that one will fail to act in accordance with accepted standards; expressions such as 'being noticed' or 'being looked at' when behaviour referred to is seen as dishonourable; and downgrading descriptions like 'little old woman'.

> (Nijhof 1995: 196)

His analysis concludes that shame for those with Parkinson's concerns 'public rule-breaking and deviance' (Nijhof 1995: 202). Non-normative adult behaviour in public, such as drooling, or messy eating, brought on by Parkinsonian symptoms, is acutely felt as socially unacceptable: social rules are broken and the protagonists branded, by themselves or by others, as deviant. Withdrawal from public life is often a consequence.

The transition from indignity to dignity, from being clumsy to graceful, albeit temporarily, is important to dance participants, and one reason they appreciate their dance classes. In a blog post for Theatre Freiburg, Anne Klausmann reflects on her dignity through dance, counteracting the dominant characterization of herself with Parkinson's as defective or deficient:

> The defect and the deficit are at the center of attention instead of the question about the possibilities even with Parkinson's disease controlling my life. How can I sustain the quality of living if I am stigmatized as a dysfunction by the diagnosis? […]. How can I keep my delight and feel like a human being, despite and besides the Parkinson's teasing […]. Dancing in the group does me good, the possibilities I see clearly, I feel my dignity, I am respected and not weary of starting again and again and of making a dive at the bright side of life. Of loving my life and myself, of caring for me and keeping me warm, of caressing my soul, of growing wings, so I can fly to my places of longing away from harm. The distance between me and the sickness gets greater, I can forget about it and suppress the thought of it to make me soft against the hardening and stiffening from outside, and I make room for change and a time out.
>
> (Klausmann 2015)

Klausmann pinpoints the double challenge to maintaining her dignity: the negative reaction of others, who see bodily dysfunction and do not understand (as in the examples above) and the medicalization of the condition, in which she is the sum of her life-changing disease. In dancing, Klausmann finds a different path that allows her to feel dignified and graceful. She uses ideas, such as caressing, wings, flying and caring to emphasize the gracefulness in feeling safe, relaxed and dignified. She may be able to step back from the overwhelming feeling of having Parkinson's and within that breathing space, alter her negative thoughts about herself.

The importance of facilitating a dance class so that participants both feel able and can witness others' capabilities, rather than their disabilities, is underscored by participants' comments. 'I watch all the waltzing and tango on *Strictly Come Dancing* [televised ballroom competition] and I feel sad because I can't do that any more, but coming here, I'm still a dancer, I still feel able' (Carroll F 2013). 'It makes you aware of the grace of your body I suppose because when you have this kind of condition, your body image is very negative […]. You can forget about the disease itself' (Desi B 2013). 'At the end, when we stood in a circle and pretended we held something in our hands which was very precious to us and passed it round the group, I found it very moving that EVERYONE in the group did this with great tenderness and care' (Dorothy S 2013). The perception of still being able, of feeling capable of taking ownership of a situation in a way that is respectful and caring to others and oneself, is crucial in the manifestation of dignity. The control and integrity of the body, seen as crucial in Chapter 5 is also important in contributing to dignified grace.

Creating a life with dignity involves possessing capabilities, which are important to many people's quality of life (Nussbaum 2007). The capabilities approach asks: 'What is each person able to do and to be?' (Nussbaum 2011: 18). This question is answered by a number of capabilities, laid out by philosopher Martha Nussbaum (2007, 2011). These capabilities include good health, bodily integrity, being able to use the senses, imagination and thought, expressing emotions, having social and political affiliation, being able to play. Being able to do something to enhance one's quality of life, however, requires having access to the means to realize it. To have capability may mean to receive extra care and/or financial support to accomplish something, as in the case of someone with a disability. A dance programme tailored for people with Parkinson's may fit into Nussbaum's definition of capabilities. Within dance for Parkinson's sessions, people are considered artists and they are able to dance, to imagine, to play, to sense their own bodies moving in relation to others, not forgetting that to enable capability may mean explicitly offering dance sessions that a person living with Parkinson's feels will be for him or her and will expressly develop dignity through those capabilities listed.

Feeling able can be supported by being respected. Grace as dignity is relational; it requires the respect of others. Henry Home, Lord Kames, who popularized the Enlightenment view of grace as dignity, defined dignity as the sense of self-worth that attracts respect from others (Sparshott 1995). But the dignity implied by Kames suggests that respect may come from prestige and honour, rather than a mutual respect for humanity. I challenge Kames' notion of grace as dignity with the Parkinson's context since social success and prestige are not of primary concern in here and indeed can be seen as contrary to community dance's notion of inclusivity.

With regards to the requirements for dignity, sociologist Richard Sennett (2003) makes a distinction between self-respect and respect from others. Craft-workers, as Sennett defines musicians and dancers, may feel self-respect – indeed, arts projects are often valued for generating self-esteem – but not necessarily mutual respect. In much of western society, Sennett reasons, respect and dignity are formulated around people's ability to take care of themselves, particularly financially by having a job. This is a difficult proposition for people with Parkinson's because few work, and a number are dependent on a carer. Sennett offers the idea of autonomy as a means of acknowledging a more reciprocal respect, which can lead to dignity. Following psychoanalyst D.W. Winnicott, he defines autonomy as 'the capacity to treat other people as different from oneself, understanding that separation gives both others and oneself autonomy' (Sennett 2003: 120). We are not required to understand the differences that separate ourselves from others, but to acknowledge and accept these differences. For autonomy to engender respect, both people must accept that their knowledge and experiences are different but not greater or inferior to those of the other person. Sennett concludes,

> Conceived in this way, autonomy is a powerful recipe for equality. Rather than an equality of understanding, a transparent equality, autonomy means accepting in the other what you do not understand, an opaque equality. In so doing, you are treating the fact of their autonomy as equal to your own. But to avoid the virtuoso's mastery, the grant must be mutual.
>
> (Sennett 2003: 122)

By 'virtuoso's mastery', Sennett means that commitment to the craft through self-respect is not a commitment to respecting another. Respect must be mutual. Sennett's argument sits within the capability approach, explained above, in the sense that the person's knowledge and experience contributes to their actual capability. While Nussbaum's argument states that good caregiving with dignity may expand the receiver's ability to express their individual knowledge and experience openly, rather than hide them from general view, Sennett's conception of autonomy relies on both parties to be sensitive enough to acknowledge each other's capabilities.

Importantly, dancer Sharon Resen observes people witnessing and respecting what others can do in the dance class, irrespective of how little that might seem. C's walk across the floor, mentioned above, allows others to witness grace and respect the dignity of his movement. This is a special event for those in the room. In watching research film footage of the English National Ballet's London class, participants were particularly struck at how their fellow dancers engaged with the movement. Comments such as 'we don't look as if we have Parkinson's. C looks so strong! M has no hesitation' and 'you are remarkably still R; I haven't seen you that still' (discussion group 2014c) underscore the supportive way that participants respond to each other's dancing. These comments suggest how mutual respect and a sense of dignity are created. In supporting the dignity of the dancer, the observer carries out a graceful action too.

These comments reveal that dignity arises from acceptance of who people are and from the connection people feel with others in the group. As Alan F (in discussion group 2014d) stated, 'it's a communal activity. We develop as a family'. As explained in Chapter 3, Wilcock and Hocking (2015) argue that 'being' and 'belonging' are essential to health and well-being and are found in valued occupations, such as dance for Parkinson's classes. Wilcock and Hocking talk about 'being' as calm acceptance of who one is. For these dancers, having Parkinson's in common plays a part in their feeling of closeness. One person expressed, 'you think you are all alone with this situation but this dancing makes you realize you're not' (Anon. 2, discussion group 2015). But as another participant points out, it is not the disease that brings people closer, but their collective development of an attitude towards the condition and towards each other:

> My attitude towards myself has changed. This is so welcoming and a non-judgemental sort of atmosphere of welcoming and acceptance, me learning and possibilities [sic]. Here we are crooked and falling over and we're allowed to do it.
>
> (Valerie, in discussion group 2015)

The non-judgemental, non-stigmatizing atmosphere, also invoked by Klausmann, embraces the participants as dancers full of possible capabilities, despite being 'crooked and falling over'. The acknowledgement of their state of being and the acceptance of their condition, but also the celebration of their potential and the witnessing of actual capabilities, creates mutual respect and dignity.

Mutual respect and dignity is important here, as the witnessing participants also acknowledge their own achievements, as well as vulnerabilities. In her work on illness in written narratives, literature and medical humanities, scholar Ann Jurecic proposes,

> Practicing acknowledgement entails recognizing the complexity of living among others, where one is always performing arts of social reading and interpretation. In contrast to knowing or judging, acknowledging also entails recognizing one's own ignorance and vulnerability, as well as the unpredictability of social encounters and relationships.
>
> (Jurecic 2012: 63)

Acknowledgement is different to judgement. Participants seek not to evaluate each other, or crave the self-important dignity as propounded by Kames. They realize that what they witness is what they feel themselves. The communal bond here is what materializes out of the mutual respect given and received.

The feeling of community in a Dance for Parkinson's class comes through strongly in the film *Capturing Grace*, partly because of the respect members give each other and through the dignity of their dance. Director of Dance for PD, David Leventhal, comments in the film,

> The bonds of community are incredibly strong. They have learned to create something that wasn't there before, a sense of joy and confidence and grace. There is a sense of dignity with […] performing and going beyond what they thought they could do.
>
> (Iverson 2014a)

The Brooklyn Parkinson Group members demonstrate that dance enables them to act with dignity. Leventhal notes they achieve a state of performance that they were not expecting to achieve with Parkinson's because the disease and social anxiety dictate the ability of that person. Instead, the dancers flourish as performers.

Participants understand the effort people make in order to dance. As Jane D'A (2010), a member of the English National Ballet London class, comments, 'it's being with people who are the same as yourself and all making every effort. Because what you're feeling yourself you know what effort they're making'. This is not grace defined wholly by physical effortlessness, but also by a rare effortlessness in how people create a humane and respectful space for each other. Jane D'A understands the effort that people with Parkinson's have to make in many areas of their lives. Yet none of the participants, still less the teaching artists, know what an individual experiences with Parkinson's. The disease is too fickle and varied for a unified experience, although each participant has a general idea of what a fellow dancer with Parkinson's goes through. In the dance space, all participants and leaders need to enact Sennett's notion of autonomy, respecting without possibly understanding. In this way, I argue, grace as dignity evokes ethical grace, whereby a human being cares for the stranger, not necessarily to understand, but to respect with dignity, his or her autonomy as a person, irrespective of whether his or her body is whole or not. The idea of ethical grace presents a different challenge to community dancers and dance teaching artists than the notions most commonly associated with dancing grace. I suggest that it is through the imagination that artists may describe this ethical grace and through imagination that we, as human actors, may take up the artists' challenge.

The ethical stance that grace demands stems from its origins in theology. For Renaissance writers, such as Castiglione, achieving grace meant moving closer to God. His imagery of the dancer's rise as symbolic of reaching the heavens clearly indicates dance's link with cultural and religious beliefs in sixteenth-century Italy. The spiritual connection of physical grace in art is the point that intersects with theological ideas, still central in Christian, Hindu, Islamic and Jewish traditions, among others. Theological concepts of grace are definitely different and separate from a secular artistic tradition (Duffy 1993),[5] but where a culture is steeped in religious custom, such as Renaissance Italy, it comes as no surprise that grace in art touches upon the threshold of theological grace.

Writing at the turn of the twenty-first century, theologian Jeannine Thyreen-Mizingou (2000) suggests that some poets deal with ethical grace as a theme in their poems, which translate divine unconditional love – the grace of God – to a human responsibility to care for one another. She argues that in postmodern times, where fundamentalist religion and other meta-narratives of the Modern era sit uncomfortably in a pluralist society, a secular grace may be cultivated in humane responses freely given to the stranger.

## Grace as gift

An ethical grace may be developed further from the notion of allowing respect and dignity to the act of giving, receiving and returning. I entitle these triplet actions 'grace as gift'. Grace as gift has its artistic and philosophical origins in the Renaissance term *gratia* (kindness, favour, gratification), described above as one of two strands of grace, the other being *venustas* (charm, loveliness, beauty). Additionally, grace in connection to gift is found in theological, sociological and humanist discourse. The gift of God's grace has a long theological history, particularly in Protestant Christianity.[6] In contrast, a Weberian sociological reading of grace extracts all links to theology and connects it to charisma (Potts 2009). As explained above, a humanist reading explains grace as unsought-for generosity to a stranger (Thyreen-Mizingou 2000).

Mindful of the Renaissance term *gratia*, philosopher Francis Sparshott argues that in touching hands, the Three Graces symbolize 'the three phases of generosity: giving, receiving, and returning' (Sparshott 1995: 461). The phases of generosity are encapsulated in the idea of gift, which is given, received and often passed on to others. I argue that for dancers with Parkinson's, generosity is the outward manifestation of grace as dignity, where that care and respect received and given to each other on the dance floor resonates out into their communities. The dignity implied by grace is evoked here and given a platform for action in the wider world.

Before exploring the ethical dimension of grace as generous gift, at this point it is worth outlining the notion that creativity and Parkinson's itself are seen as gifts and are present in many individual stories told by people with Parkinson's. These are not necessarily stories of relating to others, but they are narratives of individual expansion of creativity in people's lives. What is striking about dance participants' stories is how many acknowledge the gifts that they sense Parkinson's brings to their lives, such as a surge of creativity and a consequent interest in participating in artistic activity such as a dance class. Claims that people with Parkinson's have increased creative activity or inspiration, particularly in art forms they previously had not explored, are wide-spread. For instance, Renée A, who attends a dance class in Germany, started poetry writing prolifically, as has Danny N, a dance-participant in Israel, and Martin G, a dance-participant in the Netherlands. Eddie N from London started woodcarving after taking up dancing. Scientific research in this area is in its infancy, but studies have suggested a link between dopaminergic medication and increased productivity within arts practices, as well as increased artistic sensitivity in some individuals (Kulisevsky et al. 2009; Inzelberg 2013). One study has suggested that creativity is heightened in people who develop impulsive-compulsive traits as a result of Parkinson's medication (Joutsa et al. 2012). There is speculation that the loosening of inhibitions that often comes with Parkinson's may encourage people to take risks – to try an activity they normally would not do (such as dance), or to create an artistic work, which arguably relies on exploring ideas differently, with all the risk that that entails. Joutsa et al. (2012) caution, however, that increased practice and motivation in an artistic activity often lead to an increase in ideas, skill and perception. Thus, the special link to Parkinson's could be tenuous.

Irrespective of the possible causal nature of their augmented interest in creative pursuits, many people with Parkinson's claim that their new-found creativity is a gift. In *Capturing Grace* Reggie claims that dancing has 'liberated a part of me, a sense of creativity' (Iverson 2014a). Wilcock and Hocking (2015) argue that however it is defined, creativity constitutes a key human capability and that activities encouraging it can have 'a major impact on health and well-being' (2015: 190). It may allow people to 'bring order and meaning to their lives' (Wilcock and Hocking 2015: 244) and thus contribute to healthier living. Wilcock and Hocking describe creative activity as a capability – a 'doing' – that contributes to 'becoming' (2015: 239), that is, aspiring, achieving, developing and growing. If dancing with Parkinson's is seen first as a creative activity, and second, as an activity embedded in daily life, then it offers adherents a means of bringing order and meaning to their lives. In possessing a condition that threatens turmoil for people, the opportunity to dance regularly is a gift that develops healthier living. Beyond that, it may contribute to a sense of achievement, development and growth, rather than to a feeling of degeneration and a focus on the meaninglessness of the disease. Development, growth and achievement need not reside solely in the individual, but can radiate out to others. Dance may offer the impetus to the receiver to share with others in a way that encapsulates what dance offered them.

According to dance participants, Parkinson's develops or heightens qualities such as awareness and compassion for others and for oneself. In *Capturing Grace*, Joy from Brooklyn finds that Parkinson's 'builds patience, compassion, a sense of the human condition and it makes you reflect on what's valuable in life and in that way I'm thankful' (Iverson 2014a). Dancing acts as a means of sharing these gifts and acts itself as a gift.

After early onset of Parkinson's, Pamela Quinn gave up her career as a dancer. Yet she realized that her professional knowledge and understanding of movement helped her manage the condition in a way that not many others could. (She only started to take medication fifteen years after diagnosis). She now teaches others with Parkinson's how to use the movement ability they have to greater effect through her Movement Lab at Mark Morris Dance Center, New York. Quinn has appeared in two films as both dancer and narrator. In the film *With Grace* (Spink et al. 2013), in which she dances with David Leventhal, Quinn talks about discovering gifts:

> This disease is so hard, you say. No doubt. But in a way it gives us more of each other and it bears other unexpected gifts: creativity, empathy, lack of inhibition. What choice do I have to try to accept those gifts with grace?
>
> (Spink et al. 2013)

In *Welcome to Our World* (Bee 2010), Quinn cites patience, compassion and perseverance of spirit as three other gifts that she has received through developing Parkinson's.

The double meaning of the phrase 'with grace' becomes more potent as viewers, watching Quinn dance gracefully, are told that she has Parkinson's, a condition that is believed to take away graceful movement. But she accepts this gift with grace: grace becomes inextricably linked to the grateful, yet humble and dignified, receiving of a gift. Quinn is aware that this grace is an opportunity to tell her story through her own embodied narration.

Notably, she gives her gift of grace to others with Parkinson's as a movement teacher. One of her students writes,

> Pam, I think you are really helpful to me because you are a teacher who really cares. The fact that you also have Parkinson's disease and can move so well is truly an inspiration. Because you are a teacher who has Parkinson's disease is a tremendous benefit to the students in the class. You know exactly the correct cues to give to help us all move safely and with grace.
>
> (Tobey 2016)

Quinn describes herself as an 'outlier' (2013: 40), as someone extraordinary, who has discovered a way to keep moving in spite of Parkinson's through her knowledge and experience as a dancer. She is one of a handful of professional movement artists with Parkinson's – such as ballet master Alexander Tressor (United States) and clown Paul MacDonald (United Kingdom) – who have decided to share their unique perspectives with other people with Parkinson's.

Sharing gracefully is not purely reserved for professional artists. There are examples of community Parkinson's dancers giving back to others with care and dignity. For instance, members of the Queensland Ballet Dance for Parkinson's group in Australia raised funds for those who could not afford physical therapy to take part in solo or small dance classes regularly (Jeffrey 2016). Participants of the Weymouth dance for Parkinson's group in south-west England and their spouses regularly go away on holiday together, thereby sharing the considerable organizational stresses of travelling with Parkinson's, as well as the camaraderie.

When he first started dance for Parkinson's classes, Roy K had been fearful to face others with Parkinson's:

> About a year and a half ago I avoided getting involved in meetings with Parkinson's people. I was frightened and not wanting to admit to having Parkinson's. I overcame that. It was one of the important outcomes of this for me.
>
> (Roy K 2011)

After having been a regular dance participant for two years, he decided to set up a drop-in centre for people with Parkinson's in London, assisted by a few others from his dance group. The centre gave the opportunity for people living with Parkinson's to socialize and have a coffee break within a supportive environment. Three years on from starting dancing, he was also running a drop-in centre at a pub in London for people with Parkinson's, so that their carers could go shopping or have lunch without the added caring responsibility. Although these initiatives are not necessarily wholly because Roy K started dancing – it would be naïve to think this was the case – it is clear from Roy K himself and his fellow dance participants that these initiatives are bound up with how he and they approach life with dancing. Their approach is characterized by empathy, respect and generosity.

While community dance has largely restricted the exclusionary connotations of grace (established in the Renaissance), twenty-first century disability dance can embrace the concept of grace in a new way. I maintain that it is possible to use the concept of grace in a community dance context if the definition is expanded. Grace opens up to a new characterization that acknowledges some of the historical definitions, at the same time as translating those into the dance for Parkinson's setting. The three meanings of grace that I propose here draw upon how dancers with Parkinson's feel grace has touched them. The association starts with physical grace. In the Parkinson's context, physical grace still takes on the specialness and sense of wonder seen in the writing from Renaissance authors, yet it is not necessarily the virtuosic fluidity belonging to the professional dancer. Physical grace is an internal feeling, as well as a change in quality of movement that can be discerned from an external eye, to be specific, a quality discerned by someone who is able to know that they are seeing a change in a person's fluidity and who is affected by this observation. The act of witnessing physical grace is the first step along the way to enacting the second characterization of grace as dignity. Grace as dignity is relational, where there is care and respect for one dancer from another and from witnesses to dancers. The empathetic 'we' is implied in the connection between people, which is then expanded outside of the dance situation to grace as gift. It is a generous enactment of grace as dignity in another environment; a sharing of the quality of grace in the wider world. Grace in a dance for Parkinson's context is relational, community focused and through the moving body it emotionally connects people together.

## Notes

1   In 2014, *Capturing Grace* won the People's Choice Award at the Mill Valley Film Festival in Marin, California, and the Starz Denver Film Festival in Denver, Colorado, both in the United States.
2   The 'elite' dancer transcends the weightiness of fatigued, ungraceful movement, according to dance scholar David Michael Levin (1983). Levin sees grace as a conversation between weight and weightlessness. He argues that the great skill of a dancer (and he talks mainly of the ballet dancer) lies in his or her ability to play with the tension between showing that body has weight and disguising the body as a material object through the illusion/attempt of weightlessness. In this illusion, time and space are seemingly suspended for the viewer. He writes in relation to the qualities in the work of ballet choreographer George Balanchine: 'The syntax [of the dance] must utilize and acknowledge the tangible weight, the massive balances of the body, but only in order to defeat or suspend them, and to render the objective body as a magically weightless, optically intangible presence' (Levin 1983: 132). The dancing body is not the object of attention so much as the spectator's experience of its movement. The materiality of bone, muscle and skin and the mechanical (technical) execution of movement are superseded by the ability of the dancer to transcend these functional elements.
3   Foster (2011) gives a rich and engrossing account of the ideas of kinesthesia and empathy in dance performance through the ages, which encompasses mirror neuron theory and expands beyond it. Reynolds and Reason (2012) give a different account of kinesthetic empathy within a variety of specific creative and cultural forms, but which, again, expands beyond the mirror neuron theory. Reynolds (2012) examines the dancer's body.
4   See Renee M. Conroy (2013) for a rebuttal of this particular conclusion.
5   Theologian Stephen Duffy argues: 'There is little interplay between its [grace's] secular and theological uses. In a theological context we do not have in mind the poise of a wide receiver or a ballet dancer [...]. One might even claim that the interplay between secular and religious uses of the word "grace" are improper, for the Christian Scriptures hardly ever draw a connection between *charis* and an aesthetic quality [...]. Suffice it to say that *charis*, *gratia*, and "grace" have traveled different historical roads' (Duffy 1993: 29).
6   This book makes no attempt to grapple with the complexity of theological interpretation in this area, nor with the conflicting commentaries by theologians of different persuasions. For a critical, non-conformist analysis, read John Oman (1919), and an alternative Catholic analysis, Stephen Duffy (1993).

# Chapter 7

Finding freedom

Two lines of dancers face each other as the thumping pulse of Stravinsky's *The Rite of Spring* starts up. Marching in towards each other, the figures throw their arms upwards and sideways as the music accents the driving rhythm. Turning to face the front as they meet, the dancers march towards the audience, obeying the irregular crashes on the piano and Congo drum by whipping their arms up or down, hands splayed open. They chant, with the defining accents of the music visible in how they speak and move:

Standing here together
with the choSen one to Be with you,
the Rhythm will take Over and we'll Feel it in our boDies.

Stamping and vocalizing altogether as one group, the dancers convey the theme of sacrifice and fertility ritual within the story: collectively they must accept the Chosen One who will die to ensure the growth of their crops. Collectively they dance as one unit; as the clashing, crashing chords drive forward the movement.

(Houston field notes, Tate Britain London 2012)

The Parkinson's dancers who performed *The Rite of Spring* in 2012 at Tate Britain, one of London's most famous art galleries, did so with control, coordination and vigour. The performance was part of a residency by English National Ballet, whose version of this work (MacMillan, 1962)[1] requires dancers to pay constant attention to difficult rhythms, synchronization, unison and precise movement. At the same time, the work conveys a terrible understanding that someone is going to be killed. The dance feeds on the terrifying helplessness felt by the sacrificial victim facing the inevitability of her death. The work goes on to physically convey feelings of terrible chaos as death nears. Loss of control and chaos are two powerful feelings experienced by dancers with Parkinson's. The two features – of control and of chaos – illustrate the powerful oppositions at the heart of dancing with Parkinson's. They both are manifest when participants talk about freedom.

Through this chapter I articulate experiences of freedom in response to dancing. I explore the concept of freedom, as seen within the dance for Parkinson's context, as a series of opposing characteristics. Described by the Parkinson's dancers themselves, dancing loosens the body up so that the dancers are able to move in a more expansive, less constrained way, as well as with more risk. By contrast, dancing brings wayward movement under control – 'control' meaning the freedom to move with strength and precision. Yet the dance sessions

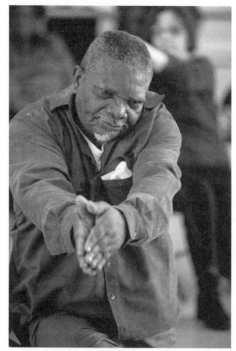

**Figure 7:** Dance for PD at Mark Morris Dance
Center, photography by Rosalie O'Connor.

are seen as places where people may be more uninhibited and less worried about non-normative behaviour. But while it is a space where people can feel more at ease with having Parkinson's, it also gives them the freedom to forget about their condition for a while. These series of contradictory characteristics mark freedom for dancers with Parkinson's.

## Freedom: Body fluidity and loosening

On one level, dance participants may conceive of freedom as a bodily experience. Margaret O describes it as a process of lubricating the body so that the experience of moving becomes more fluid:

> I'm not sure if the dancing helped me physically but it did make me move more freely and smoothly and helps a lot when meds are not working so well. The rhythm and music give a boost to start moving and then I feel less stiff and more flexible and it was easier to continue.
>
> (Margaret O, in discussion group 2013c)

In corroboration, Desi B (2013) noticed her fellow participants 'loosening up' during the sessions. Many dancers, irrespective of whether they have Parkinson's, will recognize this process within their own bodies, particularly as they age. Many dance sessions are devised to warm up the body, muscle group by muscle group, with exercises gradually building up in terms of pace and complexity so that the body has the chance to become conditioned enough to cope with bigger or more refined movement. This way of developmental working is typical of most western dance practices.

Yet, for dancers with Parkinson's, this process is more dramatic because of how the condition has affected their bodies. When Charlotte J and Paul Q talk of freedom, they are comparing their bodily abilities and sensations before and during the dance session. Charlotte J (2013) exclaims, 'it's amazing, I am running across a room. It can make me feel very free, wonderfully free. And it is wonderful to be made to move in ways that one does not normally move'. Charlotte J does not literally run across the room, but she moves more confidently, faster and with more fluidity. The freedom that she feels prompts her to describe the experience *as if* she were running: not hard graft running, but running with the wind in her hair. It is a pleasurable physical sensation, accompanied by equally pleasurable personal imagery. Paul Q (2012) echoes Charlotte J's pleasure, 'I do enjoy it so much. I am using parts of my body I don't normally use. When I leave here I've got a spring in my step. I can't put it into words how I enjoy it, but I do'. The spring in Paul Q's step is both metaphorical and literal. The bounce of his loosened body is matched with the buoyancy of his mood. With their habitual movement patterns confining the range of their movement, people with Parkinson's find liberation in moving differently.

Loosening of the body is also described as a metaphysical loosening from bondage. In talking about his need to dance when he starts stiffening up, Ray P uses the term 'break out'. Often 'break out' is used to describe escaping from prison and the ensuing liberation is often viewed as contributing to societal chaos. Ray P would not label his Parkinsonian body as a prison – he is far too optimistic for that – but the image of revelling in the freedom found through dancing is clear and characterizes Ray P's way of dancing, where he bounds around the space, moving his arms up, down and around. It is an improvised dance that generates more and more movement and exudes expansiveness. Wonderfully spontaneous and without structure, it verges on a delightful chaos. Ray P describes his frustration at not being able to talk to his neurologist about his method of escape:

My consultant doesn't say anything about it. It's disappointing he's never watched me break out. I had a student doctor once and forced him to watch [...] he said it was amazing as suddenly I'd broken free and it clicked.

(Ray P 2012a)

Ray P's frustration with his neurologist demonstrates how beneficial the dancing is to Ray P's quality of movement. Ray P dances whenever he feels he is getting stiff and wherever he may be – in the supermarket, on an aeroplane mid-flight or at a restaurant, as well as in the dance studio. He always carries an iPod with a long playlist of tracks of both classical and popular tunes, which help him move again. He prefers fast music, as he finds it easier to move to a quick tempo. Ray P dances freeform, picking up his feet, bounding, skipping and treading forwards and backwards, turning, swinging his arms and hips. He can dance for over three hours like this. He is not alone. In the film *Moving Skåne* (Hybbinette 2017), documenting the dancers who attend Skånes Dansteater's dance for Parkinson's programme in Malmö, Sweden, Georg S is seen dancing along a road with his headphones in place, whilst others walk past. Dancing is what keeps him moving and helps keep him independent.

Similarly, Pat K from London remarks of her fellow dancers that she observes a dropping away of, or escaping from, a constraint:

> In class when it gets to the point of doing walks [striding or marching across the floor], I'm not someone who changes dramatically with walks, but to look at others and see them free from something. I think of freedom when I see them.
>
> (Pat K, in discussion group 2014c)

Pat K does not feel that she 'changes' when striding out to music, which is an indication of the eclectic experience of Parkinson's. Pat K's observation of her fellow dancers suggests that they are liberated from a particular way of moving with Parkinson's, possibly free from some symptom, or from certain habitual actions and reactions, and in addition, that they look different because of this. For Pat K herself, who does not feel affected in this way, it is motivating to witness the freedom of movement in her fellow dancers. Her experience suggests that freedom of movement may be inspiring and infectious.

## Freedom through improvisation and play

The potential to move more freely is provided by specific movement structures set up within many dance for Parkinson's sessions. Dance structures, such as movement tasks and improvisation scores, which demand cooperation amongst dancers, lead to play. The importance of play in achieving freedom is observed in the improvisatory tasks in a dance session at the Kleines Haus, a theatre space in the State Theatre, Freiberg, Germany. Here dance teaching artists Clint Lutes and Gary Joplin direct a movement improvisation through a text-based score danced by Parkinson's participants and post-graduate scientists from the University of Freiburg. The score consists of a series of commands that the dancers have to carry out in the space:

> Look at a body part.
> Move it.
> Look at another body part whilst continuing to move the first.
> Put your hand on a part of the body that you cannot see.

Move that part.
Take your hand away but keep the movement of that body part in your hands.
[...]
Form two lines.
Dance.
Dance how a five year old would dance.
Do something specific but only do half of it.
Change location.
Look where you came from.
Slowly change level.
Everyone move in the same direction.
Change direction.
Again.
Again.
Take a position like an animal.
Move like it's hunting.
Slowly attack another animal.
Continue and hum a favourite song.
Exaggerate movements slowly, still singing.
Hold onto something.
[...]
Fall.
Connect with someone else.
Hold that contact point and move the rest of the body around this point.
Stop and disconnect.
Reconnect.
Disconnect.
Reconnect.
Stay connected but change location.
Continue but form one group.
Altogether without speaking form the shape of a giant boat.
Smile.
Finish.

(Lutes 2015)

During the session, dancers move alone and together, playing through movement with the images they conjure up from the score. Their movements are funny, serious, silly, big, small, unusual and collaborative. Participants are given the freedom to interpret the facilitator's prompts as they wish. As the group travels on an exploratory movement journey, many non-verbal questions are negotiated physically, individually and collaboratively. Imagination, both through directed imagery and spontaneous emergence, fosters new movement shapes and qualities. Improvisations directed by a score, a set of instructions, can encourage dancers to move purposefully away from initiating a particular movement in a habitual manner. In other words, the instructions given allow the dancers to circumnavigate unconscious patterns of regular initiation, progression and accomplishment of movement, but in a playful manner.

For Batson et al. (2016), the aim of improvisation is 'to stimulate new pathways for motor learning by meeting unexpected environmental conditions arising in the moment and devising new physical solutions as a result' (Batson et al. 2016: 6). They suggest that the quickness of cues, or instructions, helps participants to make immediate decisions to move beyond their 'self-perceived capability' (Batson et al. 2016: 6). Moreover, the multi-tasking inherent in many instructions guides the dancers to move in non-habitual patterns, freeing up the body to experience new ways of moving. As Chapter 3 points out, people with Parkinson's often fall into very pronounced habitual ways of moving within a narrow range of movement qualities and trajectories. Moving within these confines can lead more readily to unstable situations and falls, as the body is less prepared to improvise around a situation of imbalance. We need the freedom to act differently in order to navigate a risky environment.

Disorder is risky, even dangerous. To arrive at the dance class, particularly by public transportation, participants have to risk travelling. They may have to cope with potential falls, with potential freezing, with disparaging remarks from passers-by. For some, this takes confidence; as Carroll F explains,

> You loose a lot of freedom with this disease. At one stage I was afraid of leaving the house. I was afraid of falling down. I started to be afraid all the time [...]. Coming here I have a sense of freedom that I can move and share with others who have the disease. I go out now. I'm still afraid, but I know I can do it.
>
> (Carroll F, in discussion group 2014d)

Pat K, Mary C and Margaret P tell of travelling from the English National Ballet class on the London Underground. Whilst on the escalator, Mary C lost her balance and fell, pushing Pat K, Margaret P and others over. The risk of losing balance is high when negotiating waves of crowds, moving vehicles and escalators. In response to these risks, teaching artist Ann Dickie (2010) created an exercise for her London group of Parkinson's dancers, at their request. It recreates the criss-crossing, variable flow of people at Waterloo station, a major railway and Underground terminal, in order that they could practice body awareness skills and interrupted flow of movement in a safe environment. The relative social safety of the dancing environment means that participants may feel more able to practice risky movement.[2] The 'Cappuccino' command in the Dance Well class – instructing participants to stand on one leg – is an example of this. The command is not, 'Stand on one leg!', but an image irrelevant to that act. The irrelevance tricks the brain into performing an act that the participants may have assumed they could not do, or were too scared to try. The association between fear and action is lost in linking the unconnected image to the instruction and then to the action.

Using a different explanation, dance scholar Danielle Goldman points out that the 'disorientation' offered in an improvisatory setting, where fixed, known points of reference are uprooted, is an engagement with difference – be it physical, cultural or political – and allows dancers 'to make something creative' (Goldman 2010: 54). She implies that dance improvisation has uses beyond the studio and her ideas have resonance for people with Parkinson's. In her case studies, in which dancers improvise a negotiation with political, social, physical and cultural 'tight spaces', Goldman argues:

> At its core, improvisation demands an ongoing interaction with shifting tight places, whether created by power relations, social norms, aesthetic traditions, or physical technique. Improvised dance literally involves giving shape to oneself and deciding how to move in relation to an unsteady landscape. To go about this endeavor with a sense of confidence and possibility is a powerful way to inhabit one's body and interact with the world.
>
> (Goldman 2010: 146)

From Goldman's stance, the Freiburg score can be seen as a starting point to think through the 'tight space' in the 'unsteady landscape' that Parkinson's creates. Improvisation, Goldman argues, is a powerful tool in dealing with constraints because it is 'characterized by both flexibility and perpetual readiness' (Goldman 2010: 5). It challenges 'expectations of fixity' (Caines and Heble 2015: 3). Deliberately asking someone to change direction, when changing direction is often fraught with challenge, or to move part of the body that may not have felt movement for a while, both recognizes the tight space and pushes dancers beyond it. The Freiburg score offers avenues of exploration that widen movement possibility when Parkinsonian habits may often close down that freedom. It offers a safe, yet expanding space to explore challenging movement and stiff bodies. In exploring those tight spaces, the tightness may become slacker.

## Freedom to control movement

Control over one's movements, realized through focused action, is an act of will (Fraleigh 1987). Movement control gives the performer the freedom of choice of where and how to project his or her body in space. This choice is not always open to people with Parkinson's, as they often do not have control over their movement. Dyskinetic, dystonic or tremulous movement forces them to move against their will, and bradykinesia causes them to move at a pace which is not necessarily of their choosing, disrupting or preventing sequential or multiple movements from being performed. Through dancing, many people with Parkinson's may experience a freedom of choice because they gain some degree of control over their actions whilst in a musically charged and facilitated space. This space differs from the public space, where they must negotiate unforeseen objects and situations and cannot count on awareness of or concession to vulnerability. It also differs from the domestic space, where the support needed to facilitate 'getting out of trouble' is not necessarily available. Freedom of choice is controlled by stabilizing muscles and through proprioceptive, intentioned actions. I argue that it elicits a feeling of emancipation to revel in a moment of control.

Dance scholar Sondra Fraleigh (1987) argues that dance is an activity in which skill and control can lead to the freedom inherent in the mastery of actions. Following the philosophy of Paul Ricoeur (2007), she suggests that creating and practising movement through an act of intentional will can lead to mastery over movement so that it becomes unconscious and involuntary: 'I must exercise my will, but in the final analysis, I seek to move free of effort and wilfulness. I seek to move freely, spontaneously, or in total accord with the will' (Fraleigh 1987: 19). Ricoeur (2007) argues that our bodily actions possess a tension between voluntary (intentioned) and involuntary (habitual, unconscious) movement. He maintains that habitual actions are at once intentioned and unconscious. We have mastered the will over muscular effort to produce involuntary movement. He concludes, '[t]hrough habit I take possession of my body, as the words *habere, habitude*, themselves suggest' (Ricoeur 2007: 315). Fraleigh is concerned with professional dancers, who, after many years of practice to hone skills, reach the stage where their mastery of the body allows them to concentrate on performing, rather than on executing a step, which now comes 'naturally' to them.

For people with Parkinson's, however, the normal tension between voluntary and involuntary movement is broken. The basal ganglia of the brain, where dopamine is produced, controls voluntary movement. With a depletion of dopamine, the ability to initiate movement – in other words, the 'doing' moment after choosing to act – is compromised. Conversely, involuntary movement (including hypokinetic states) increases. Parkinson's is a counterpoint to Ricoeur's beautifully crafted thesis. Voluntary movement requires effort, but cannot cross over into involuntary habit. Parkinson's symptoms, not the will, are in danger of 'taking possession' of the body.

Learning how to control movement frees dancers from some Parkinson's limitations. Many dance for Parkinson's classes still follow the technical tricks inherent in exercises to strengthen, lengthen and stabilize the body in order to accomplish dynamic movements, such as large, fast, whole body movements, with ease and accuracy. For example, in Rotterdam, the Dance for Health class participants are invited to 'talk' with their backs when opening their arms out, becoming aware of the stabilizing scapulae against the ribs, whilst in London the English National Ballet class participants are given the image of wearing a corset or suit of armour to think about engaging the muscles of the abdomen. Imagery, used in these examples to help stabilize the torso, is complemented by other techniques, such as using strong, physical dynamics to lengthen the body's reach and to practice stabilization whilst moving. Conscious use of eye focus helps create movement that is intentional and purposeful, helping to control movement. DAPpers (Dance for the Ageing Population), the dance group for those with and without Parkinson's in Providence, Rhode Island, United States, exhibits all these elements while performing the movement vocabulary of American modern dance choreographer David Parsons. Slashing their arms through the air to the right above their heads and then back across their bodies to point downwards to the left, the dancers take on the fast, complex cross-rhythms of the music to emphasize its strong accents. Their heads turn to look at their hands, as their arms cut through the air. The use of strong musical and physical dynamics in this instance allows participants to practise gesturing with focus and intention.

A group from English National Ballet's London class demonstrates that practising control gives the illusion that the dancers are not affected by Parkinson's. When observing film footage of themselves dancing, the participants commented on this:

> It looks as if we're supposed to be doing that. We're not lost anywhere.
>
> It looks slick, really good.
>
> We look like we know what we're doing. As our disease progresses we are gaining skills.
> (English National Ballet discussion group 2014c)

The group noticed the intention and clarity of the movement, as well as the diminishing of obvious Parkinsonian movement. In other words, through control of where and how the actions of the body are performed, freedom of movement may flourish. Intention and direction are just as pertinent as physical mobility to controlling movement.

In observing Dance for Parkinson's beginner 'taster' classes[3] next to the regular class at English National Ballet, it is noticeable that Parkinson's dancers with more experience pick up spatial patterns and movement sequences quicker than those new to the class. This observation suggests that the ability to retain and develop skill often remains – other parts of the brain are also used in this task (Calvo-Merino et al. 2006) – but neurologically the challenge remains of making that voluntary movement habitual and involuntary. Since action-making with Parkinson's often involves thought and effort in order to accomplish movements, the achievement of freedom that is spoken of amongst dancers with Parkinson's may be linked more to motivation,[4] effort and dance knowledge than to the mastery of movement.

## Social freedom

Although control over movement may give people the freedom to initiate and focus gestures and steps, the class is also a place where participants need not feel inhibited by their Parkinson's symptoms, providing another kind of freedom. Alan F (in discussion group 2014d) remarks, 'I come here and I feel I can shake at will and not worry about it and not feel cast out [...]. I come here and feel relaxed'. In the class, he does not feel embarrassed, worried about, or stigmatized for his tremor and dyskinesia. Disability and dance performance scholar Petra Kuppers summarizes the companionship offered through dancing with others with disabilities: 'A lot of disabled dancers I know are glad for the opportunity to dance with other dancers to whom different forms of embodiment are not strange, but familiar in their individual strangeness. There is so much less explanation necessary' (Kuppers 2011: 2). Alan

F does not have to explain why he is shaking, or moving in the uncontrolled way he sometimes does. People within the dance class accept his way of moving, even if they do not have the same dyskinesia or tremor. He thus enjoys a social freedom within the class setting.

Similarly, Carroll F (in discussion group 2014d) describes the dance session as a social space and time where she, as a person, takes priority over her condition: 'I find my friends who don't have Parkinson's want to ask about my illness and fuss over me so I don't see them often. Here I can be myself'. Kuppers again concurs: 'Physically integrated dance environments are havens for many of us, places where we can be free to explore who we are' (Kuppers 2011: 2). Disorder is welcomed and valued as part of the class; it is not a problem that must be addressed. The fact that symptoms may lessen during class is a pleasant addition to the experience, but not essential to the operation of the programme, or to participating.

This attitude, cultivated by teaching artists and embraced by participants, can be construed as subversive, particularly by a society that makes assumptions about who can dance. The valuing of atypical ways of moving within a space reserved for the mastery of movement and performance within specific cultural frameworks, in the case of English National Ballet, the Mark Morris Dance Group and Queensland Ballet, for example, can be seen as a reconfiguring of the assumed purpose and users of these hallowed studios. In dance for Parkinson's classes, a space traditionally earmarked for rehearsing control of the body is used in a manner that allows for disorder and lack of control, and is much less stringent than the ethos of traditional dance classes. The classes inhabit an arena where even the smallest, or most uncontrolled, movement is valued as a contribution to the widening patina of bodily action and where individual interpretations of themes from company repertory are celebrated. Dorethea from the English National Ballet London programme explained:

> It frees you up. It freed me up. I'm a bit self-conscious as I'm not doing it right and I'm the only new person there […]. When I first started I was thinking was I doing it right? Then I threw myself into it. It was fun. It was doing something different with no one looking at you.
> (Dorethea 2012)

The lack of inhibition that Dorethea experienced contributes to the sense of carefree disorder within a space. The irony is that this same space is where professional dancers rehearsed beforehand and have wept after hours of gruelling effort to achieve perfection.

Carroll F (in discussion group 2014a) remarks: 'I find it liberating. I can make a fool of myself and no one cares'. Like Carroll F's use of 'fool' when commenting on the carefree attitude of fellow class participants, Ann Klausmann, a member of the Freiburg dance for Parkinson's class, uses the related term 'jester':

> For me it will rain red roses, wonders and miracles to meet […] I have the jester's license to broaden my horizon. I am alive, here and now, I no longer conform, me and my body are transformed – that allows me to behave outside of what is fitting and of what is safe.
> (Klausmann 2015)

The 'fool' is someone who does not conform, whose appearance and behaviour is idiosyncratic, who laughs, who resides on the margins and who plays with the tension between order and disorder (Ran 2007). The dance session becomes the playground where the jester is granted freedom to act, or say, what others cannot, or do not. Parkinson's disrupts the normative order of action, use of space and traditions of the dance studio. Dancers with Parkinson's could be conceived of as residing on the margins of dance culture, mostly unseen as performers and yet present as dancers (Grace 2009), and as straddling the border of movement order and disorder. They often do not conform to mainstream bodily action, and have great capacity for laughter.

Laughter can be the outward expression of subversive freedom. Carroll F (2012b) confides that the class 'allows us to laugh at ourselves. Privately I call us The Tremblies'. This type of humour also is seen in the name of the Parkinson's blog written by dance advocate Kate Kelsall, Shake, Rattle and Roll (Kelsall 2014).[5] Carroll F's subversive humour can be seen as part of her experience of identifying with the group of dancers, but in a way that dislocates the group from being passive consumers of a dance product. On these terms, the group becomes a troupe, 'The Tremblies', players who actively reposition themselves from consumers to performance-makers. Carroll F plays disruptively with the idea that the aim of participation in cultural activity by those with a neurological disorder is to help the dancers get better, and that the participants ought to be grateful, compliant sufferers of a serious disease. Dance for Parkinson's is not about getting better, nor is it about being grateful, but about discovering the delight of dancing within an artistic context. The concept of the 'fool' stirs up what is expected and assumed, which further frees up thinking on how participation in dance can be approached.

Some people with Parkinson's identify themselves through labels such as 'Parkie'. They appropriate names that subvert the serious intention of the disease, allowing them to create a positive identity around their condition. Although only privately voiced, 'The Tremblies' acts in the same way. Kuppers (2011), who identifies herself as disabled, points out that words to describe disability often have long histories across different cultures and languages; some of these words have contributed to oppression and stigma. She suggests that one of the approaches to highlight 'the non-fit of language and lived reality, is to mark the play we can engage in with words, within and across languages' (Kuppers 2011: 23). Taking the word 'cripple' as an example of a word that has simultaneously signified uselessness and oppression, as well as power and celebration of disability within the genre of crip poetry, Kuppers relishes in the resonances, both physical and metaphorical, that the word gives to her:

'Cripple' is so much richer than 'disabled' as a sound, as an image, bound to a longer heritage [...]. Rejected trash becomes an object of beauty, moving in its own gravity.

(Kuppers 2011: 25)

The reclamation of words and movement with new histories is forged within art and actions of disabled artists. 'Queer' terminology is another example of repossessing language (see, for example, Livia and Hall 1997 or Croft 2017), and community dancers are no exception to this alternative action. In playing freely with expectations, taboos and assumptions, people marginalized through labels may find new expressions of identity. In creating a place where difference is embraced, such as the dance for Parkinson's class, I maintain that it may create a fertile place for that freedom of expression and the freedom to take on a positive identity.

## Freedom from disease

Dance for Parkinson's sessions offer participants a period of time when disease is not the focus. Pat K (in discussion group 2014d) says, 'the focus of the activity is on art, not Parkinson's. I don't think about Parkinson's from beginning to end. I don't think "this is good for me" during class, doing steps, doing it for Parkinson's'. Dancing can open up the world, just as Parkinson's can close it down. A participant from the Queensland Ballet Dance for Parkinson's class says, 'I felt free. I didn't feel I had anything hanging over me. Quite hard to explain it. But I did things that I normally wouldn't have done. And that's very important' (Participant A cited in Jeffery 2014a: 14). Freedom in forgetting the drudgery of dealing with Parkinson's is important to people who have to manage a complicated medication regime, wayward symptoms and changing conception of selfhood. Sally B and Margaret O also find that dancing can unlock this freedom. Sally B exclaims, 'the most noteworthy thing is that we forget that we have Parkinson's', to which Margaret O responds, 'yes, we get carried away with it' (Sally B and Margaret O, in discussion group 2013b). Desi B suggests that forgetting is a positive action:

> Everyone is kind of in the same position. You're not the odd one out. I can imagine people are very aware of people watching them in a negative way, whereas this is much more positive. You can forget about the disease itself.
>
> (Desi B 2013)

For Desi B and many of her fellow dancers, the focus on the process and joy of dancing is a distraction from the daily grind imposed by their medical condition and from any suffering they endure.

## Freedom to transcend

For others, dancing may allow people to forget, or transcend their condition by finding a new freedom of expression through movement. In a poem he wrote, Martin Giling, a participant at Dance for Health, Rotterdam, explains how dancing, as an outlet for expression, permits him freedom.

'The Dancer: A Hidden Strength'

Searching for the light
reaching, moving out, probing…
stretching his limbs
Beyond time and space
the past is forever more present,
hidden within the folds
of his own fabric
a secret, even to himself.

Everything is interlaced,
locked from within.
Fighting for freedom of expression
and self-motivated interest
he releases,
from deep within himself,
a hidden strength,
never known before.

Moving forward,
leaping ahead,
discovering the dancer, within his own life.
Sensing and sharing his strength
with all those who care,
listen and respond
to the infinite possibilities of growth.

(Giling 2015)

Through dancing, freedom from thinking about Parkinson's opens out the world again. It can straighten out the chaos often instigated by the initial diagnosis. In a magazine interview Giling explains: 'It was a black page in my life. I had a lot of trouble accepting it [Parkinson's diagnosis], was apathetic for a long time. I could not rid myself of the thought that my life was over' (Giling 2014: 37). Giling goes on to claim: 'When I dance, I feel like a different man. My whole being, my whole life opens up onto the dance floor' (2014: 39). Straightening out the chaos means increasing the possibilities of action and interaction. For Giling, dancing, as an embodied practice, enlarges perspective again, often whilst sharing movement and bodily experience with others. The witnessing and sharing of his body's rhythms, textures, scars and pleasures with others viscerally shapes chaos into narrative. Giling crafts his body into one that can speak clearly again and move with others. 'The creativity and playfulness inherent in dance, I feel, are unique […]. Plus the fact that you are always working within a group, encouraging each other, creating something together. Now that means a lot to me. I also see other people gaining a lot from it' (2014: 39). Importantly for him, this act allows for growth in terms of nurturing a positive new identity as a person with Parkinson's. Giling perceives the dance group as a place where, in growing together, people with Parkinson's might find freedom from their daunting diagnoses and begin to chart new journeys.

Giling's poem reflects Arthur Frank's recommendation for 'the *need* of ill people to tell their stories, in order to construct new maps and new perceptions of their relationships to the world' (Frank 2013: 3, original emphasis). Dancing with Parkinson's foregrounds the disease – these bodies are scarred with its effects – but in creating their own movement patterns, styles and stories, dancers start to form wordless personal narratives. Although Frank focuses on the verbal telling of stories, he proposes that stories are also embodied. The dancing stories are not necessarily about suffering. Participants may witness suffering within each other's bodies, but the dancing stories are also infused with joy. Opening out into the world happens for them through joyful dancing.

Frank further suggests that stories help to validate the presence of the teller through the listener. A listener gives the teller the weighty, embodied presence to push against the 'horror' (Frank 2013: 112) of chaos, to create light and growth out of a place where the self is nowhere and nothing. Dancing with others and allowing others to watch are dance's translation of the listener and teller, or as in Giling's poem, the dancer and the responder. Giling's 'searching for the light' invokes dancing as a lifeline, a way out from being 'locked from within'. The embodied expression of the self also 'disassembles' (Frank 2013: 144) the medical story of the person as patient, a story in which the body is seen as locked, or in deficit. Frank argues that 'medicine as scientific, professional activity can only recognize the body as carrier of disease' (Frank 2013: 144). Dancing opens the possibilities of conceiving of the self because it gives the protagonist the chance of expressing his or herself differently to the patient-self. This opening out into the world is a valued freedom.

I contend that freedom for dancers with Parkinson's encompasses several elements, some of which may seem contradictory. Some of those elements are to do with physical freedom: loosening up in order to move freely, controlling muscles and developing control over intention and purpose through movement. Dancing allows for the practice of freedom, of training the body to be flexible in 'tight spaces', to take on risk in order to be safer. Although grounded in the dance event, other elements focus on the social and cognitive: freedom for dancers with Parkinson's also means having social freedom from judgement and assumptions about how a person with Parkinson's should act. Dance also acts as a distraction from thinking about Parkinson's. This freedom allows dancers to develop self-expression through movement. It is this freedom of expression that allows dancers with Parkinson's to think differently about their relationship to disease. In the next chapter I move forward with this idea to investigate the effects of freedom of expression on developing agency for the dancer.

## Notes

1   In 2017 English National Ballet reproduced Pina Bausch's version of *The Rite of Spring* and again, the Parkinson's dancers explored the theme and work in their classes. The rehearsal

director of *Rite* for Tanztheater Wuppertal, founded by Bausch, gave a workshop for the group, signifying the importance of the art within the programme.

2   Within Dance for Parkinson's sessions, teaching artists enforce safe practice protocols. These do not preclude some risky movement being facilitated, but ensure that other safeguards are in place so that participants may practise safely. This may mean pairing the least stable with dance session helpers, for example.

3   'Taster' classes are one off classes where you can sample – taste – what it is like to participate before making a commitment to attend regularly.

4   Apathy is a common behaviour associated with Parkinson's (Dujardin and Defebvre 2012), and so personal motivation is important to enable a person with Parkinson's to move. Although dancing can help bring control and focus to movement, it is the motivational aspect of the class that makes moving easier. The high adherence to dance sessions testifies to participants' motivation to attend regularly despite having to negotiate crowded public transport systems, unreliable taxi services and days when bodies are not responding well to medication (Hackney and Earhart 2009; Earhart 2009; Batson 2010; Houston and McGill 2013).

5   Other general Parkinson's blogs, which typify the humour are, for instance, Twitchy Woman (Krischer 2016) and Shaky Paws Grampa (Hall 2015).

# Chapter 8

Understanding agency

In his diary, Michael B wrote a short chapter about his life dancing with Parkinson's. His thoughts wandered from cricket, to his ballet class, to his family and back to cricket again. Within his writing, he gave little indication of any physical benefits of dancing, but he did offer the thought that dancing allowed him to get 'Mr. Parkinson out of the driving seat of my life' (Michael B 2011). In this wonderfully evocative soundbite, Michael B provides the suggestion, echoed by many, that dancing offers a way of maintaining or developing a sense of agency and identity that is neither overruled, nor dictated, by Parkinson's.

Agency is commonly defined as a state of control over one's life. Personal agency is the self-actualizing capacity to act on one's own behalf and meet one's own needs, freely and without coercion. In order to have agency, the commonly held assumption is that an individual must be allowed to make rational, productive decisions (see, for example, Leighton 2009). In addition, the agentic individual is normally thought of as autonomous: he or she can work alone. The agentic person is thus celebrated as powerful because he or she is not only able to make decisions productively, but also is a free agent.

I explore and problematize this notion of agency, seeking a different characterization that takes into account what I observe happening in the dance for Parkinson's context. I relate agency to how a person (perhaps frail, or getting frailer) chooses to live a life with dance as a key emotional and imaginative component. I argue that relationships and the environment play key parts in how people cultivate agency through dance. Notably, this chapter examines the physical environment as an emotional touchstone, as well as how people's engagement with movement may relate to their own choice in how to live with Parkinson's by creating a style of living.

## Agency in older age or ill health

The idea of agency may become particularly challenging for those faced with long-term degenerative illness or loss, particularly because these strike as people age. Biological ageing is seen as a problem in many, particularly, western, societies. The medical and societal challenges associated with ageing are separated from issues concerning other (younger) adults, and as a consequence, they are seen as detached from the concerns of the broader population. Ageing becomes then – not a function of the lifespan – but rather, a societal (and therefore medical) problem (Baars and Phillipson 2014). Moreover, the problem is seen as not ageing itself, but the *person* who is ageing and thus he or she is seen to have

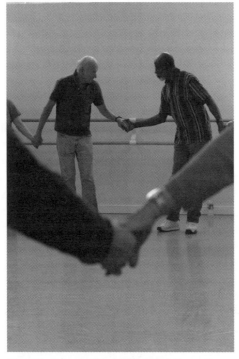

**Figure 8:** Dance for PD at Mark Morris Dance Center, photography by Amber Star Merkens.

greater need to rely on welfare, medical services and on others. This assumption negatively affects perception (of others and self-perception) of how much agency the person has, or is expected to have. Parkinson's can be seen as a specific example of accelerated ageing (Solimeo 2009), where a diagnosis can prompt people to feel negatively that their bodies and life course are beyond their control. Solimeo finds that Parkinson's

> is a disorder whose early symptoms bear a striking resemblance to widely held models of normal older age, [which] presents a unique and thought-provoking case study through which we can examine how culture comes to bear on the experience of the body and ultimately, how older adults' embodiment reflects and produces aging as a parade of unavoidable losses.
>
> (Solimeo 2009: 6)

People may feel vulnerable or alone, if they have experienced, for example, the recent loss of a partner and/or the onset of a medical condition, particularly if they are without a strong social network. They may feel that they have decreasing opportunities to forge their lives how they would like.

The connection of agency with autonomy is perhaps more idealistic than realistic, however. As social gerontologists Jan Baars and Chris Phillipson note, '[s]eemingly independent individuals are in their daily lives not only continuously dependent on activities of others but also confronted with systemic forces beyond their control' (2014: 14). In other words, those who feel they have ownership over their decisions in life may have a network of support in order to function in this manner. Even those who have a secure support network may come up against barriers to autonomy, such as ill health. Autonomy is always precarious and reliant on others to develop and so the agentic individual is only partially, but never fully, autonomous. To achieve agency, an individual needs to be connected to others. Sociologists Anja Machielse and Roelof Hortulanus (2014) point out the more resilience and social competencies people build up over their lives, the less challenging vulnerable situations are. They assert that well-being is greater if people find a balance between independence and support from, or connectedness to, others. They argue, '[i]t is precisely in a life phase in which people are confronted more often with radical life changes […] that self-confidence and self-respect are important' (Machielse and Hortulanus 2014: 121). Parkinson's is a condition where symptoms can easily undermine self-confidence, particularly in socializing and meeting people. Chapters 1, 5 and 6 give examples of the Parkinson's dancers' networks shrinking, as disease becomes more noticeable and more interfering with social engagement.

Agency is not just partial, relying on the support of others and having the potential to be battered by ill health, it is also locally determined, being recognized and defined by the local context in which the person lives, for instance, his or her geographical and social environment and the available support. Social gerontologists Jaber Gubrium and James Holstein define agency as 'both the provision of, and responses to, reasons for why […] people have done what they did, why they act as they do, who they conceive themselves to be, and what they might do in the future' (1995: 556). Agency may therefore be characterized as being the way we mark our own identities. Gubrium and Holstein argue that agency may be found in the mundane, everyday tasks and cultural artefacts that surround us and that create meaning within our lives. I would add that the inclusion of others within those local contexts enriches the possibility of agency (and take it away, should those others be domineering or bullying). And so in defining agency, I would add to Gubrium and Holstein's list by asking: with and for whom does the individual act at any specific point in time and place? People, as well as artefacts, may colour and deepen meaning in our lives.

The environment and relationships play particularly important roles in the establishment, or maintenance of agency. These roles are particularly acute in a situation where an older person might be characterized as a 'fourth ager', where he or she has severe impairment and is frail. For fourth agers, the definition of agency needs to be reconceived to take into account more subtle expressions of will and of identity, which depend upon the level of support the person has (Grenier and Phillipson 2014). If the frail older person has help to communicate and act, his or her needs and wishes are more likely to be met and agency is more likely to be maintained. People's experience of local contexts, including environmental, social and support factors, conditions individual expressions of agency, particularly when focusing on fourth agers, as agency is fashioned by the experience of the culturally embodied person, his or her environment and his or her relationships. Local contexts do not either straightforwardly open up autonomy, or close it down, but rely on an exchange between the person, his or her environment and relationships, which are felt as meaningful. Personal background can frame agency through locally shared meanings (the communal), biographical particulars (the personal) and material objects (the physical) (Gubrium and Holstein 1995). I would add, it also happens within shared practices, such as dancing, that hold value for participants. Bearing in mind shared meanings and practices, the personal and the physical, I argue that agency becomes an environmental state of being.[1]

## Places of the heart

A sense of connection and communal belonging may spring from an environment in which a body of action is discovered, explored, developed, practised and, notably, loved. Dance scholar Judith Hamera describes this environment as an 'affective geography', where place is physical, but also 'of the heart' (Hamera 2007: 69). Hamera highlights the ballet studio as one place where attachment is nurtured through the act of dancing, specifically, through the technique of bodywork prescribed by the tradition of classical ballet. In her study of a ballet studio in Los Angeles and the young people who attend class there, Hamera argues that the place is transformed, yet anchored, by the codified action and rituals of the moving bodies in the space. Without the collective tradition of movement that connects the young people, the studio is merely a shabby brick building with no particular significance. In other words, a place of the heart is called into life by the traces inscribed and formed by moving, interacting bodies and people.

At English National Ballet in London, the studio echoes with the real and imagined traces of professional ballet dancers rehearsing. The real traces – such as the practice tutu left in the corner, the bottle of water by the *barre*, the smell of sweat and the humidity of the room, the casual, turned-out walk of the dancer, clothed in woollens, who gives a shy smile as she passes through – are joined by the unseen and imagined: the circular traces of pirouettes in the centre of the floor, the swish of legs at the *barre*, the charged tension of the *pas de deux*. These real bodily inscriptions are joined by symbolic ones: the beauty and glamour of the ballet dancer at the peak of condition, the technical honing of the moving body that signifies quality, the live music that underscores the allure and quality of that performance.

For many of those attending the Parkinson's class, these real and imagined traces are part of the lure of dancing. Alan F (in discussion group 2014d) exclaims, 'you get a sense of occasion coming to this venue. It heightens the experience [...] it's so uplifting for me'. He contrasts the English National Ballet class with the Parkinson's support group that meets in a care home, where he feels negativity bound up with, for him, the symbolic stagnation of the body and mind. Cultural studies scholar Sonjah Stanley Niaah, in her examination of Jamaican dancehall, names 'performance geography' as including 'the ways in which people living in particular locations give those locations identity through certain acts' (Niaah 2010: 32). Similarly, Alan F performs a positive emotional and physical act in dancing in a location that connects him to an identity that is not bound up in the drab, undignified grind of Parkinsonian degeneration. Not only does the dance studio give him a sense of aliveness through the youthful and vibrant traces left by professional dancers, but the prestige of the location is important to his experience. Alan F compares it to playing at Wembley, the international football stadium in London that is home to the England football team: 'By coming here it's a bit like going to play at Wembley. It's so special. It's like going out on pitch and training at Wembley' (Alan F, in discussion group 2014d). The magic and glamour of the association with professionals at the top of their career are key to the specialness. Alan F (in discussion group 2014d) notes that his friends are 'fascinated that I am training with English National Ballet'. In the way that he talks about his dance for Parkinson's class, allowing the symbolic association to filter through his conception of the programme, Alan F is acknowledging his sense of attachment and belonging to the ballet institution.

Sometimes imagining its past creates the specialness of a space. Being in the same place as others who have inhabited the place, fashioning history through their movement, can be rousing. As theatre designer Iain Mackintosh remarks, spaces where people have performed house 'ghosts from the past' (Mackintosh 1993: 86). Whether in a theatre, church or munitions factory, past rituals of moving leave traces that can build excitement for the present inhabitants because of the histories and/or tradition that they invoke. Mackintosh notes 'the buzz' that audiences can receive from entering a theatre space (Mackintosh 1993: 86). Spaces are inhabited, given life and shared across past and present through movement.

In evoking its specialness, it is possible to conceive of the dance studio as a quasi-sacred space, set apart or marked out from other spaces (Eliade 1959). To dance (or, to 'act') within this special environment can be viewed as a ritualistic practice, where a specific way of acting differentiates the practice from other, more everyday activities and, therefore, these actions create an aura of specialness and meaningfulness for participants (Bell 2009). Anthropologist Catherine Bell argues that physical actions within ritual practices create an embodied identification with those practices and their meanings. She writes, '[t]he act of kneeling does not so much communicate a message about subordination as it generates a body identified with subordination […]. For all intents and purposes, kneeling produces a subordinated kneeler in and through the act itself' (Bell 2009: 99). In the case of Alan F, the ritual act of taking ballet class creates identification with the glamour, vitality and precision of moving that the ballet company exudes. The act of dancing in this environment produces an embodied feeling of being not only a dancer, but part of the specialness that English National Ballet exudes.

Those with Parkinson's who dance in Bassano del Grappa's civic museum echo Alan F's identification with the specialness of the dancing place, because the galleries are brought to life in the imagination of the dancers. Surrounded by the paintings by Bassano's foremost Mannerist painter, Jacopo da Ponte, Eva B remarks on how dancing there contributes to the quality of her life:

Dance makes me feel beautiful. Dance gave me back a sense of harmony which I thought I'd lost [...]. I feel God dancing with us. Indeed, dancing next to the paintings of Jacopo da Ponte is like being inside the Bible itself! I am aware that all these emotions combined together change the quality of your life. If I close my eyes, I'm still able to see all the paintings around me and all the movements too.

(Eva B cited in Cinconze 2015)

The paintings are large – figures in reds, pinks and oranges stretch upward towards the ceiling. Framed in dark gold, they bring a reverence to the large, vaulted room. Kneeling, genuflecting, pleading, striding, playing, praying, sewing, fishing, the figures are dynamic. It is as if they accompany the dancers as they improvise in pairs and as a group. Sometimes the movements of the dancers fleetingly echo the poses in the paintings, creating dynamic conversations between the paintings and the dancers. For Eva B, the sense of stepping in time and into time with these characters comes through her within the generous space of the civic museum. Importantly, in dancing in a space where the spiritual can be contemplated, Eva B's body executes a shift from being primarily Parkinsonian to being a part of the artistic homage to a biblical story. Her body is 'restructured' (Bell 2009: 99) through her act of dancing in the gallery environment. Just as Niaah argues that the dancehall provides 'another space, process and means of connecting to a higher self, that which is elevated beyond the drudgery of survival' (Niaah 2010: 116), so Eva B's dance for Parkinson's class provides another space, process and means of connecting to an identity and a body that rises above Parkinson's and the everyday toil of dealing with the condition.

## Agency through self-invention

The imagination that is grounded through movement has a part to play in developing connection between people. Those who dance in community halls may not feel the grandeur of the museum, or have the glamour of professional dance life entwining with their own dance experience. Nonetheless, they create their own, shared heritage of action where the movement they create together in the space and the conviviality they may share are part of developing a place of the heart. What the lowly community hall illustrates is how an unobstructed space may bring people together face to face, body to body, imagination to imagination; one where people can directly relate to each other within a space, where it is a delight to move together. To reiterate, a place of the heart is made by people, more than bricks and mortar. The institution may add to this, as seen above, but the actual movement in the space and the imaginative approaches that open up freedom of expression are crucial in developing connection and belonging. Josephine DG dances at the Old Fire Station in Oxford, a converted fire station with a collection of studios, a theatre and a café. In her diary, the movement and stories created through group tasks are the main subjects, rather than the building, or her teachers from English National Ballet, although she speaks with admiration for the latter. In one passage, she describes a simple improvised group task that demonstrates the interweaving of imagination, storytelling, movement expression and bonhomie:

> The class's version of 'Pass the Parcel' was illuminating too. We first did this a few weeks ago, all standing round the edge of the studio, receiving from the person in front of us, and passing on to the person behind, a present, which could be whatever we decided it was, different in size and weight and shape when we passed it on from when we had received it. We played it again this week. I would not have believed we could have come so far in such a short time. Everyone's movements were much freer, more individual and more exaggerated, we were much more inventive and had more confidence, and it was more obvious what more of the presents were. I got down on the floor to wrap a jumper, and tried to show how much difficulty I had in tying a ribbon in a bow. I felt I had done it rather clumsily, but to my surprise three people came to me afterwards and said how well I'd done the mime. At least, two of them did. The third, J said Christmas must be chaos in my house if I really wrapped parcels like that! (It is.)
>
> (Josephine DG 2013)

In another diary entry, Josephine DG describes the connection that dancing stories gives:

> Through ballet dancing we are no longer just people. The music carries us beyond ourselves to a world of the imagination in which we are all parts of a larger whole, not just individuals, but united in telling the elemental story of the Sleeping Beauty.
>
> (Josephine DG 2013)

Josephine DG's conception of going beyond individuals to collective story-making is a recognition of how imaginative creation may bring a sense of togetherness. Story-making may be a positive affirmation of a self that communes with the physical world and it can also allow that self to step into the imaginative realm. The group of people collectively seeking to give bodily presence to these stories counteract the physical or mental limitations that each individual may sense in his- or herself. Entering an imaginative world together creates a space for opening up possibilities for each individual and is an example of productive and powerful interdependence.

The imagination is part of dancing and part of the act of movement interpretation. Josephine DG's experience is significant to her partly because she brings her imagination into play, creating another layer of participation. Hamera argues that the imagination is central to creating a place of the heart for her group of pre-professional ballet dancers in Los Angeles. Each brought excitement and motivation to their dancing lives in the ballet studio by imagining their mastery of the technical demands of ballet, as well as their aspiration to become artists. Codified traditions of movement, such as ballet, are bolstered by an imaginative life created by those who dance. Hamera writes,

Overlaid onto, and hidden within, the rigidity of the technique is a complex geography of fantasies: dreams of physical and social virtuosity shot through with longing for an autonomous agency that both masters and exceeds technique.

(Hamera 2007: 69)

Hamera illustrates that embodying a movement practice is not just about the technical formation of the body, but also about enlarging the approach to dance through the imagination: professional and community dancers alike may do this. In this mixture of emotion and tradition of physicality, dancers move beyond their chosen movement form. In dancing, participants create affective responses to that movement practice and to those around them.

Furthermore, dance movement does not fade away once it has been performed (Hamera 2007). It lives on within the imagination of its participants and within the group of people who share the dance space and its resonances, as seen, for example, in Alan F's delight in talking about his dance class. I contend that dancing is theirs through their imaginative engagement, building relationships, developing senses of belonging and cultivating a mode of living beyond or beside their bodily dysfunction. By opening out into the imaginative lives of participants, dance becomes 'a series of tactics for living, not simply a strategy for moving' (Hamera 2007: 209). As a cultural event moulded by its participants in the way that it is imagined and adopted, dance for Parkinson's becomes integrated into how participants craft their lives. Symbolically (and so in the imagination), dancing stands for a positive, pro-active attitude to life and practically, it gives Parkinson's dancers a style by which to anchor their approach to life. Through channelling a distinctive bodily expression, the dancer embraces a style. Needing the imagination along with movement to be realized, the style lives within body expression and, further, within a life-style cultivated in response to, but not dictated by, a chronic health condition. For example, the literary critic Anatole Broyard, upon hearing he had prostate cancer, took up tap dancing. He describes this as 'evolving a strategy for my illness' (Broyard 1992: Part 2, para 36 [e-book]). He created a style, for his illness: a light-hearted foray into tap dancing. Tap dancing was Broyard's symbol of nonchalance, and a physical manifestation of pleasure. Broyard argues, 'Only by insisting on your style can you keep from falling out of love with yourself as the illness attempts to diminish or disfigure you' (Broyard 1992: Part 2, para 37 [e-book]). The movement learnt through tap classes became the embodied and symbolic stance that filtered into Broyard's approach to living with his illness, just as dancing with da Ponte's paintings became Eva B's way of enriching her imaginative and spiritual life in the face of Parkinson's and choosing to dance rather than fill in a survey became Marc Vlemmix's mode of living well (see Chapter 3).

Styles of moving can be a basis from which to characterize individual and collective approaches to living, and creating one's own style may give agency. One's own style of moving may encompass the consciously creative use of culturally embodied gestures. French literature and dance scholar Carrie Noland (2009) argues that gestures, such as those practised as dancing, can be embodied and used in unconventional ways. Gestures, as cultural traditions, are subconsciously ingrained in our bodies, but the dancer may also subvert those traditions through a conscious use of gesture. This conscious use of gesture, Noland stresses, gives the person agency. Noland asserts that just as embodiment is the 'process whereby collective behaviors and beliefs, acquired through acculturation, are rendered individual and "lived" at the level of the body' (Noland 2009: 9), so agency is the 'power to alter acquired behaviors and beliefs for purposes that may be reactive (resistant) or collaborative (innovative) in kind' (Noland 2009: 9). As shown in Chapter 7, subversion to normative uses and conceptions of moving are apparent in some Dance for Parkinson's classes. But subversion may not be necessarily what is practised. For example, although technique feeds individuals and groups imaginatively and symbolically, the ballet dancers within Hamera's study strive to model their movement on an idealized conception of technique. In other words, their aim is to conform to the technical style taught within the dance studio. Although modelling movement may not necessarily give the dancers agency, how each person uses, or how collectively they use that style, might be. Their non-conformity, or rather, individuality, lies within the 'complex geography' of fantasy, talk and longing (Hamera 2007: 69). The same may be said of individuals within Dance for Parkinson's classes. They try to align their movement along the lines demonstrated by the dance teaching artist, or, apply themselves to the task set by the teaching artist. Personal stories, ideas and images sculpt the experience as distinctive and meaningful in a way that merely aping movement will not be.

To give an example of remodelling of a technique, in Kentish Town, London, musician Anna Gillespie commissioned teaching artist Danielle Teale to lead a series of sessions for her Parkinson's dance group. Teale structured three linked exercises based on the classical ballet principle of an open, outward-facing body. The principle cultivates a body stance in which all movement emanates out from the vertical axis of the body. The upright posture is enhanced by the turned-out position of the hips, which not only opens out the pelvic region, the knees and the feet, but also elongates the line of the leg down into the floor. The anchoring of the scapulae against the back encourages the upright line of the spine to reach up, at the same time as moving the shoulders back and causing the trunk to operate in a vertical position. As a consequence, the arms reach out further and the head rotates freely on the top of the neck. The openness continues with an outward, projected gaze to an audience and movement that presents spatially in a forward and outwards motion towards that audience. In this way, classical ballet can be seen as a generous technique that gives itself, via its openness, to its spectator.

In the Parkinson's dance sessions, Teale played with the idea of open and closed, and what opening up and closing in felt like: is that an empowering movement? Is it too revealing? In this first exercise, she used the concept of public and private to consider the idea of open and closed. She took the image of the Hollywood star getting ready to go to the Oscars, as a fun way of exploring bodily the notion of private to public. Her next exercise asked participants to consider what private and public meant to them and helped them explore their own identity. They improvised around the two concepts looking at their private versus public worlds, their real versus imaginary worlds, and themselves as a person versus themselves as a person with Parkinson's. In the final exercise, Teale allowed them to improvise freely, exploring open and closed in their own way. This series of related exercises illustrates how ballet principles can be configured atypically, where the movement becomes less of an imposed technique and more of an offer to the dancers to create their own approach to thinking about the principle of openness.

## Communicative movement

Although *Dancing with Parkinson's* has discussed the effect of dancing on the individual within the context of group work, this chapter has started to develop ideas about interdependent agency as an element of dance for Parkinson's and one that operates on emotional and imaginative levels through connection and belonging. In this section, I explore how the feelings of community and solidarity might link to this conception of agency through, what sociologist Arthur Frank (2013) terms, the communicative body. Frank suggests that the recognition and acceptance of the body's contingency, its fragile, unpredictable nature, allows one to empathize with others in pain. Despite each person's pain being individual, it is possible to recognize one's own body-story in someone else's and theirs in one's own. Frank calls this open state as belonging to a communicative body, a body that has stepped beyond chaos to recognize a way of living with chronic illness. In developing an empathetic stance, he argues, the person aims to cultivate a shared sense of corporeality where he or she desires to be there for another in pain. In other words, the communicative body is formed through its relation to others. Despite participants being at different emotional stages in their individual journeys with Parkinson's, there may be instances – flashes – within the dance class where bodies align, feeling their shared corporeality. A body story is not verbal, but reveals itself and communes 'in touch, in tone, in facial expression and gestural attitude, and in breath' (Frank 2013: 49). In an earlier development of the idea, Frank (1991) suggests that people who give or receive care and those who dance develop communicative bodies. An improvisatory task in the English National Ballet London class reveals some of these communicative bodies:

> The flute meanders in and out of the couples' dancing. It is improvising around a Debussy score. It layers a lazily seductive tone to the non-verbal conversations that are being created. It is a mirroring improvisation, where one participant follows the creative dance of his or her partner. Jane N swirls her hips, flicking her hands around her husband. Mike A rolls his head to follow with his nose the finger of Jenny Harrington, one of the professional dancers joining the class. He holds onto the *barre* as he is unsteady today, but his gaze is directed towards the younger dancer. Mary C and Christine B create their conversation around a *port de bras* where their arms open wide and high. Meanwhile,

John H presses the palms of his hands to Ray P's; eyes are serious and they pause, enjoying the intensity of the moment.

(Houston field notes, English National Ballet London 2011)

In a group activity that is both physical and emotional, it is perhaps not surprising to find instances when dancing with a chronic health condition ceases to be about individual expression and becomes a vehicle for sharing in a way that is defined by empathy.[2]

There is one task that many of the dance for Parkinson's programmes use at the end of every class, including English National Ballet and Dance for PD. Josephine DG describes a version of it above. She calls it pass the parcel. More commonly, each person in turn gives a squeeze of the hand or nod of the head to say 'thank you for dancing with me' to the next person in the circle. It is a community version of the ballet *reverence*, a bow or curtsy and acknowledgement of respect. It ends with everyone holding hands and taking a bow. Fleur Derbyshire-Fox, director of engagement at English National Ballet, explains that the circle task creates connection among the dancers:

> When you're teaching, one point, actually in the circle, there is a wave that comes through you out of nowhere. I want to cry. Not such a wave of happiness, just some physical emotion passing through. It's a great feeling of connection and empathy. You have to check yourself and centre and ground yourself because you need to carry on.

(Derbyshire-Fox 2013)

The circle task is a powerfully emotional point in the session when participants are brought together, each person seeing everyone else, to share movement and the stories described through movement. Michael B (2011) notes in his diary: 'The closing circle was very moving on the 22nd – somehow we were drawn together by our disability, the only time in the class that when I felt Parkinson's really having a defining influence on the class'. Michael B indicates that this moment of facing everyone is also one of acknowledgement and openness. In that openness, the materiality of each body is exposed, but also celebrated. The circle task is notable for its warmth between people, for the laughter it generates and for the creative ideas that sometimes pass between participants and grow as they do so.

For many in dance for Parkinson's classes, the feeling of togetherness is strong because dancing offers a way of connecting with, to use Frank's words, another 'wounded storyteller' (Frank 2013). Yet this connection is within a context where imagination and fantasy play a role in allowing participants to step out of structure to create their own significant pathways, attachments and tactics for living with Parkinson's:

> All the dancers wrap around the perimeter of the studio creating a large circle. Two are seated, the rest stand, all hand in hand. Kate Hartley, the teaching artist relays the idea: pass a present round to your neighbour, thanking them for the time shared dancing. The piano and flute are ready to interact, creating a soundscape for each, individual response.

161

This is the section of the class that is repeated each week and participants are ready, a few even deciding what to do beforehand. The first few dancers turn and grip the hands of their neighbour, their heads bending towards each other in a smiling acknowledgement. But soon, the action begins to get bigger, more inventive. Someone drops the present, another staggers under its weight, another blows it across to his neighbour as if it were as light as a feather. The mime gets still more and more elaborate. Giggles abound when one woman pretends to unzip her dress and step out of it towards her gleeful male neighbour. One person receives a real kiss. When everyone has received his or her present the teaching artist throws her present up into the air to be caught by each person. They then all join hands again to take a communal bow, raising arms up. Then down.

(Houston field notes, English National Ballet Oxford 2013)

The feeling of togetherness or solidarity is accompanied by individual styles and approaches, which carry meaning and significance for each participant. David Clark (1973) argues for the need for both solidarity and significance amongst members of a group in order for a sense of community to be manifest. Clark's notion of solidarity relies upon 'all those sentiments which draw people together (sympathy, courtesy, gratitude, trust and so on), a river into which many tributaries flow' (Clark 1973: 404). Relying on several sentiments reflects the sense that solidarity can be produced in different ways depending on the context. For Clark, the important element is that people feel that they can play a part in the group activity; they need to feel significant. Clark argues that significance comes through playing a role in the group, and this must be accompanied by a sense of togetherness. I would argue that playing a role might be as little as choosing to attend and taking part. Particularly for some with Parkinson's, the act of deciding to get out of the house and participate is momentous, and sometimes the effect of making this decision is heady. Additionally, although solidarity and significance may not necessarily imply empathy for another, this definition of community has scope to allow for such a mode of communication. It might be that the significance of belonging to the dance class springs from the act of witnessing another's story, or sharing one's own. These acts, as Frank suggests, may precipitate the development of empathy and a communicative body, which may underscore a sense of solidarity. Moreover, combining these two feelings suggests that the development of community might also encourage a sense of agency on the part of the group members. They do not passively belong to a community, but feel they take part to create that sense of belonging.

The powerful resonances that Derbyshire-Fox and Michael B, as well as others, describe do not, however, necessarily last throughout the class, nor is everyone affected by them. Neither Frank nor Clark imply that solidarity, significance or empathy create deep and lasting bonds between people. As the dance class is only one activity during a person's week, it is important to note that it cannot constitute more than a fluid and transient community. Dancing offers an interesting perspective on community and agency because it is voluntary and occasional. One has to step in and out of the event and carry on with other activities.

The idea that the dance for Parkinson's sessions are part of the flow of other activities, yet marked out as special, is a take on the notion of a ritualized practice. Anthropologist Catherine Bell argues that it is important to 'look to how and why a person acts so as to give some activities a privileged status vis-à-vis others' (Bell 2009: 74) and so mark them out as special. But ascribing a privileged position to the dance class is not necessarily to make it a regular occurrence.

In her study of Irish set dancing, Barbara O'Connor (1997) also discovered that to acquire social significance the class did not have to require deep commitment and lasting bonds of friendship. In analysing her interviews with participants, O'Connor finds noteworthy

> the importance attached to friendliness, openness and inclusivity which generate a sense of belonging and security and the simultaneous acknowledgement that it doesn't have the constraints of a 'regular' community. It is sufficient to know people superficially, in fact, that is the attraction – the creation of an ephemeral and instant community which is based on voluntary association and personal choice.
>
> (O'Connor 1997: 156)

The dance class encourages a conception of community that celebrates its voluntary and occasional nature. It is a community that is created and treasured for its moment in time in the dance studio. Philosopher Adriana Cavarero (1997) argues for a definition of community that underscores group members' actual experience with each other, that appears only in the present moment of meeting: 'the group has its only reality in the *actual* and existential context of appearance, which can be renewed but not conserved' (Cavarero 1997: 23, original emphasis). She proposes an active role of community where it happens 'here and now, within the space of the actual relationship' and because of this, the temporal and spatial context becomes important for the relationships between people (Cavarero 1997: 22).

As with Frank, Cavarero emphasizes the materiality of connection: Frank champions bodily communication, Cavarero the space and time through which the body moves. Such material connection may be seen in dance for Parkinson's tasks, such as marching across the room:

> In London the music starts to build, changing to a syncopated 6/8 rhythm. The dancers on cue start to march and swing their arms moving into two lines at either side of the studio. Two walk towards each other, heels striking into the ground on the beat. They meet, greet and turn, striding out towards one of the volunteers standing, and one of the participants sitting, at the other end of the room. They are followed by other couples. Each greeting is different: some smile and incline their heads, others slap each other's hands in a 'high five', some bow to each other and some strike a pose. Some try to out-do each other in how energetically they can walk up the room – it's a brisk pace set by the musicians and the dancers swing their arms vigorously – one man even bounds down, leaping his way past others. Some walk more gently, a few link arms with a dance artist

to tread slowly but happily up the aisle. All smile, have their heads lifted, as those waiting for their turn clap along to the beat, whooping encouragement.

(Houston field notes, English National Ballet London 2014)

Within this moment, there is communication between people of varying abilities. It is a time to show off one's own style of moving and be supported by others to do that within a specific space and time – marching time and class time.

Another example of the connection of bodies communicating within the same space brings out the internal rhythms of dancers moving and passing them on to one another. In Freiburg, dance artists Matan Zamir and Nicola Mascia led a session for the Parkinson's dancers and post-graduate scientists in a large dance studio on the top floor of the State Theatre. I joined in this workshop. Zamir and Mascia asked us to move, guided by the sensations felt in our bodies, rather than by any form made with our moving bodies (such as the marching in the previous example). We were asked to 'look inwards', to attend to those sensations, closing our eyes, but soon we were instructed to open our eyes and meet those of our fellow dancers as we started to walk slowly around the studio. Although throughout the two hours we attended to the sensations we could feel at that moment, the session focused on relating outwards to others. For example, in one task we worked in pairs, reflecting the sensation of our partner's touch within our own movement. We then held onto the essence of this movement as we separated and began moving alone.

> Pairing up with a tall, stooped man with Parkinson's, I feel first heaviness in touching his forearm and hand, but there's also lightness in his touch. I try to embody these conflicting qualities. As we move around, our eyes closed, feeling each other's weight and touch, I sense a feather-light delicateness in his hands. It is a caring, even loving, sort of sensation, as if he is giving me a rose whose petals are about to fall. I then feel tremor come from his arm up through mine and heaviness intrudes again. As we separate I attempt to keep this multitude of sensations within how I move, playing with my centre of gravity. I am then instructed to pass on this movement to someone else I meet in the room.
>
> (Houston field notes, Theatre Freiburg 2015)

This task illustrates that through dance we may listen to and acknowledge each other's presence, attending to the physical sensations of our partner and passing on the resonance of his or her bodily story of that moment. In exploring movement through tasks, such as the one described above, Zamir and Mascia ask us to encounter and explore the communicative, living body of another and ourselves.

The idea of the material, physical connection and context being key to the relationships that constitute a community chimes strongly with the notion, set out earlier in this chapter, of the contextual nature of person agency. To recap, as an environmental state of being, agency relies on interpersonal relationships and local contextual factors. Having agency is bound up in how people, places and objects local to us give us the ability to choose how to act and create meaning within our lives. What happens in the present local context influences whether a person feels alienated, connected or agentic.[3] The dance tasks outlined above open up the dancers' imaginations through their bodily connections to each other. They have choices in how to act and they produce movement ideas in response to one another. Witnessing, even attempting to embody, another's movement with all its weight, flow, spatial pathways and temporal rhythms, highlights body stories – communicative bodies – and recognizes that Parkinson's dancers have partially fashioned a style for living with a chronic condition.

Yet, as noted above, dancing leaves traces. Participants create imagined and symbolic meanings from past and present dance places, dancing people and related objects. Writing about theatre, James Thompson argues that affects 'linger' (2009: 157) sometimes long after the product of the play has finished.

> The quality of the experience is not only reliant on, or reducible to, the presence of the actors on stage. Anyone who has met the joy of young people off-stage, after finishing a play, must know that their effervescence is real in the moment and no less intense because the object, their on-stage performance has passed. The play is not there anymore but the force of affect continues dynamically – and dismissing performance as ephemeral in this context seems to disparage these children's delight.
>
> (Thompson 2009: 157)

As Gubrium and Holstein (1995) argue, agency is partly created out of the actors' interplay with significant objects and localities, which sustains them. So although community may only be temporary within the confines of the actual meeting of dance participants, some of the basis of connection and of agency supported by that connection lies within the broader imaginative landscape created by each group member. This landscape may stretch into the past, as well as the present and future.

## Social participation

The creation of connection and agency through dancing also may expand outwards away from the dance event and into other activities. For some dance for Parkinson's members, dancing precipitates increased social participation, or different ways of participating socially. Although some were involved in many social activities and initiatives before they started dancing, for others, joining the dance group acted as a catalyst for their greater involvement in activities outside class. Increased social participation is seen across many dance groups in different countries. Social participation is one of the three pillars recommended by the World Health Organization for assessing the extent of functioning, disability and health in a person[4] (WHO 2002) and McGill et al. (2015) argue that it is important to examine social participation as a key indicator of impact in dance for Parkinson's classes.

For some, greater social participation lies in a greater interest in participating in cultural activities or events. Foster et al. (2013) note that participation in an Argentine tango programme for people with Parkinson's in St. Louis, Missouri, United States, led to much greater participation in low-demand activities, such as table games, reading, cooking and watching films, compared to those not dancing. Elsewhere, others have set up cultural activities stemming from friendships made within the dance class and a shared interest in participation in the arts. For example, a couple of participants from English National Ballet's Oxford pilot class decided it was too far from their home in Banbury. Because they enjoyed dancing so much, they set up another dance class closer to home. They asked English National Ballet to be involved, and the company played a role in providing live music for the class once a month and inviting participants to the theatre trips. One member of the local Parkinson's support group who is a trained dance teaching artist became the lead facilitator. Meanwhile in London, a cluster of dance participants from the English National Ballet class decided to form a singing group and asked a well-known singing teacher working with people with Parkinson's to lead them once a fortnight. Nic Ephgrave, the Central London Information and Support Worker for Parkinson's UK, affirms, 'Some people may see each other at a monthly support group and say hello, but because of the intimacy of dance, real friendships have developed, more so than with any other support group I'm involved with' (Ephgrave cited in Dean 2013: 21). Ephgrave is certain that several of the activities that the group does would not have happened without the power of the dancing to give the participants the confidence and motivation to collaborate together (Ephgrave, in discussion group 2014c).

In San Francisco, California, United States, Herb Heinz was inspired by a one-off dance session led by David Leventhal from Dance for PD to co-found PD Active. Heinz had been a member of a US-wide network for people with young onset Parkinson's, but travelling to meetings got harder and he wanted to connect with people locally. He decided to set up an arts organization as a way of meeting local people with Parkinson's. PD Active established a creative community where dance was the catalyst for offering around a dozen activities, including yoga, drumming and writing poetry. Heinz says, 'For me, to create a community so beautiful speaks to what we need. It changed my life, no doubt about it […]. Everything I do – social contact, physical activity and creativity – it's all there in the dance' (Heinz 2015). Heinz mentions other activities, such as gardening and cycling, but he returns to dance as the activity that has empowered him and the local Parkinson's community to find a way of living, which is more about care and creativity. 'The choice is isolation and dying or being helpful to each other […]. It's about empowerment that we can bring a piece of the puzzle in taking care of ourselves' (Heinz 2015).

The initiatives by Parkinson's dancers outlined above have an ethical dimension, in that they are more about helping fellow people with Parkinson's than oneself. Recognition of others' and one's own situation has led to action. People with Parkinson's find themselves in a situation not of their own making, but some limitations can be overcome through mutual support. It is the recognition of the importance of interdependence that spurred the leaders of these initiatives into action. Personal agency can be seen in how these Parkinson's dancers augmented and refined their approach to living well with their condition. Personal agency is the other dimension to the notion of grace as gift, as laid out in Chapter 6. In these instances, dance, as an emotionally resonant activity, was the catalyst for taking the initiative to reach out to others in similar circumstances.

Personal agency is always contextual, contingent and interdependent and the Parkinson's dancers illustrate why even those not typically cast as agentic might have agency. On one level, Parkinson's remains a meaningless degenerative biological condition, and 'only our response can give these situations some meaning' (Baars and Phillipson 2014: 27). Thompson finds that it is precisely through participatory art that an awareness of another's plight might develop and a meaningful response to suffering might be initiated.

> It may be, appropriately, [that] the focus for participants is painful issues in their lives or broader issues of oppression in their community. In this case, attention to delight, beauty or joy, as an integrated or preparatory aspect of the work, can awaken individuals to each other's needs and perspectives.
>
> (Thompson 2009: 170)

Not that pain must always be the focus, and indeed for the dance for Parkinson's programmes, pain is rarely a featured topic. The awareness to other's needs and perspectives as attested by Thompson is drawn out through the communicative body in the dance class. For some, this has been the turning point to act. In being drawn to support fellow people with Parkinson's, the dance participants above have created initiatives with significance for them and others. Dancing has been a physical and emotional catalyst to forging significance from having the disease through solidarity with others who bear similar challenges.

Throughout *Dancing with Parkinson's* dance participants living with Parkinson's have shown how dancing carries significance for them. The specialness of dance goes beyond being a physical activity to reach people on an emotional, empathetic level, but always, the fact that dance is a movement-based art is essential to this reaction. Through attending to the aesthetic qualities of movement, Parkinson's dancers are able to find a new relationship to their own bodies and so to their lives, which otherwise may be held hostage by the disease. Although dance may stay an individual pursuit – as exemplified by Canadian 'Parky' blogger Bob Dawson (2014), who danced to rock music in his sitting room[5] – dancing also allows for a social, physical and emotional connection to others within group classes and beyond. Dance, as a movement-based aesthetic, imaginative and communal practice, has the power to create positive impact on people's lives. In the words of Oxford Parkinson's dancer Jim S,

> I've identified about eight or ten words to describe what we're doing: imagination, creativity, language, colour, music, rhythm. And I've not come across anything, anything in my diverse life, which combines all those things. The breadth and depth of what is going on […] is significant.
>
> (Jim S 2013)

## Notes

1 Similar ideas also may be found within the writing of sociologist Pierre Boudieu (1980) in his work on habitus, where the individual is shaping and is shaped by their social surroundings.

2 It should be noted, however, that empathy may not happen instantly as it can be a terrifying experience to be newly diagnosed and encounter people in the dance class whose disease is more progressed. As I mention above, one may see brief instances where empathy may happen because people are in different emotional places.

3 In the age of the Internet, I do not discount local context as 'global', but my focus is on dancing as a face-to-face activity.

4 The other two being body function and structure, and daily activity.

5 Although in blogging about his experience of dancing in his sitting room, Dawson enabled it not to be an isolated individual pursuit, but a connected activity.

# Epilogue: A beginning

In 2016, when this epilogue was written, the phenomenon of dance for Parkinson's continues to grow and develop beyond its early stages. Its development suggests that dance for Parkinson's is not a short-lived experiment and what this book has done is to describe the genesis of a movement. The approach to facilitation and teaching dancing for people living with Parkinson's is already changing, and being thought about differently:

- A debate is beginning as to whether the term 'dance for Parkinson's' is the best name to use to describe this specialist dance provision. A dance practice *for* people living with Parkinson's may sound paternalistic. It does not take into account the fact that some of these dance initiatives are *by* people with Parkinson's and that dancing is not offered as a treatment *for* Parkinson's. Perhaps in the future the phrase 'dance for Parkinson's' will seem a dated expression, albeit not a dated practice.
- The number and type of dance forms and approaches to dance offered to people with Parkinson's are expanding. Moreover, the artistic agenda promoted by organizations, such as the Dance for Parkinson's Partnership UK, Dance Well Italy and DaPoPa France, is seeing a broader and more diverse mix of dance artists sharing their artistic and community practices in the dance for Parkinson's context. This has the effect of widening artistic, movement and cultural approaches to dancing with Parkinson's.
- As noted in Chapter 2, People Dancing and Dance for PD in a joint initiative have instigated online training for dance teaching artists new to facilitating dance for Parkinson's sessions, to reinforce and enhance face-to-face training programmes in the United Kingdom, United States, Canada and Australia. It is likely that other countries and organizations will follow suit and that online training, and perhaps digital teaching (such as in Dance for PD's DVD programmes and Hamilton City Ballet's digital 'at home' programme), will become commonplace.
- A few doctors are prescribing dancing for their patients with Parkinson's. If more medical professionals become convinced of the benefits, prescribing dance may become more conventional.
- Partnerships are starting to emerge, and in the future, these may become the glue to help sustain dance for Parkinson's practice. There could be partnerships between dance and health organizations, dance and social welfare organizations, dance organizations and health insurance companies, dance organizations/artists and higher education and vocational institutes, as well as between dance companies and other more strategic arts organizations, or indeed between dance companies and independent artists and local, small-scale arts organizations.

These examples suggest that my account of the dance for Parkinson's phenomenon does not end with the publication of this book. In fact, this is an account of the *beginning* of the dance for Parkinson's movement, the founding of a specialist dance practice.

It is also a beginning for some of the individuals and groups who dance. As this book has highlighted, the desire to go beyond being a patient with Parkinson's has been palpable. The quest to find a style of living with the condition has taken people on a journey to and even beyond dance. As such, it will be difficult to predict how the dancers themselves might develop the practice of dancing in the future. That is an exciting thought. The idea of opening out a practice through the ideas, desires and inspiration of participants themselves takes dance for Parkinson's on its own journey of artistic development, grassroots action and joyful collaboration.

# Bibliography

Acocella, Joan (1998), 'Mark Morris: The body and what it means', in A. Carter (ed.), *The Routledge Dance Studies Reader*, London: Routledge, pp. 269–77.

Adamovich, S. V., Berkinbilt, M. B., Hening, W., Sage, J. and Poizner, H. (2001), 'The interaction of visual and proprioceptive inputs in pointing to actual and remembered targets in Parkinson's disease', *Neuroscience*, 104:4, pp. 1027–41.

Akroyd, Sue (1996), 'Community dance and society', in C. Jones (ed.), *Thinking Aloud: In Search of a Framework for Community Dance*, Leicester: Foundation for Community Dance, pp. 17–20.

Armstrong, John (2004), *The Secret Power of Beauty: Why Happiness Is in the Eye of the Beholder*, London: Allen Lane.

Arnstein, Sherry R. (1969), 'A ladder of citizen participation', *Journal of the American Institute of Planners*, 35:4, pp. 216–24.

Arts Council England (2017), 'Our mission and strategy', http://www.artscouncil.org.uk/about-us/our-mission-and-strategy. Accessed 6 January 2017.

Ashcroft, Bill (2001), *Post-Colonial Transformation*, London: Routledge.

Association of Dance Movement Psychotherapy (2015), 'Home', http://www.admt.org.uk. Accessed 9 August 2015.

Baars, Jan and Phillipson, Chris (2014), 'Connecting meaning with social structure: Theoretical foundations', in J. Baars, J. Dohmen, A. Grenier and C. Phillipson (eds), *Ageing, Meaning and Social Structure*, Bristol: Policy Press, pp. 11–30.

Banes, Sally (1987), *Terpischore in Sneakers: Postmodern Dance*, Middletown, CT: Wesleyan University Press.

—— (2000), '"A new kind of beauty": From classicism to Karole Armitage's early ballets', in P. Z. Brand (ed.), *Beauty Matters*, Bloomington, IN: Indiana University Press, pp. 266–88.

Bartlett, Ken (2008), 'Love difference: Why is diversity important in community dance?', in D. Amans (ed.), *An Introduction to Community Dance Practice*, Basingstoke: Palgrave Macmillan, pp. 39–42.

Batson, Glenna (2010), 'Feasibility of an intensive trial of modern dance for adults with Parkinson disease', *Complementary Health Practice Review*, 15, pp. 65–83.

Batson, Glenna, Hugenschmidt, Christina E. and Soriano, Christina T. (2016), 'Verbal auditory cueing of improvisational dance: A proposed method for training agency in Parkinson's disease',

*Frontiers in Neurology*, 7:15, https://www.ncbi.nlm.nih.gov/pmc/articles/PMC4756105/. Accessed 24 February 2016.

Batson, Glenna with Wilson, Margaret (2014), *Body and Mind in Motion: Dance and Neuroscience in Conversation*, Bristol: Intellect.

Beckley, Bill and Shapiro, David (eds) (1998), *Uncontrollable Beauty: Towards a New Aesthetics*, New York: Allworth Communications.

Bee, David (2008), *Why Dance for Parkinson's Disease?*, Mark Morris Dance Group and Brooklyn Parkinson Group, http://markmorrisdancegroup.org/resources/media/2performances/11whydancefor-pd. Accessed 20 October 2009.

—— (2010), *Welcome to Our World*, https://pdmovementlab.com/art/. Accessed 31 October 2017.

Belfiore, Eleonora and Bennett, Oliver (2008), *The Social Impact of the Arts: An Intellectual History*, Basingstoke: Palgrave Macmillan.

Bell, Catherine (2009), *Ritual Theory, Ritual Practice*, Oxford: Oxford University Press.

Benjamin, Adam (2002), *Making an Entrance: Theory and Practice for Disabled and Non-Disabled Dancers*, London: Routledge.

Bergson, Henri (1910), *Time and Free Will: An Essay on the Immediate Data of Consciousness* (trans. F. L. Pogson), London: George Allen and Unwin.

Bessing, Wyatt (2008), 'Balance and freedom: Dancing in from the margins of disability', in N. Jackson and T. Shapiro-Phim (eds), *Dance, Human Rights and Social Justice: Dignity in Motion*, Lanham, MD: Scarecrow Press, pp. 285–87.

Betarbet, Ranjita, Sherer, Tod B., MacKenzie, Gillian, Garcia-Ousna, Monica, Panov, Alexander V. and Greenamyre, Timothy J. (2000), 'Chronic systemic pesticide exposure reproduces features of Parkinson's disease', *Nature Neuroscience*, 3, pp. 1301–06.

Bishop, Claire (2012), *Artificial Hells: Participatory Arts and the Politics of Spectatorship*, London: Verso.

Blasis, Carlo ([1820] 1968), *An Elementary Treatise upon the Theory and Practice of the Art of Dancing* (trans. M. Stewart Evans), New York: Dover Publications.

Bourdieu, Pierre (1980), *The Logic of Practice* (trans. R. Nice), Cambridge, MA: Polity Press.

Brand, Peg Zelgin (1999), 'Beauty matters', *The Journal of Aesthetics and Art Criticism*, 57:1, pp. 1–10.

—— (2000), *Beauty Matters*, Bloomington, IN: Indiana University Press.

Brandstetter, Gabriele (2005), 'The Code of Terpsichore: The dance theory of Carlo Blasis – Mechanics as the matrix of grace', *Topoi*, 24, pp. 67–79.

Briginshaw, Valerie (2009), *Dance, Space and Subjectivity*, Basingstoke: Palgrave Macmillan.

Brinson, Peter and Crisp, Clement (1970), *Ballet for All*, London: Pan Books.

British Heart Foundation National Centre for Physical Activity and Health (2009), *Active for Later Life: Making the Case for Physical Activity and Older People*, London: British Heart Foundation, http://www.bhfactive.org.uk/older-adults-resources-and-publicationsitem/99/index.html. Accessed 19 December 2014.

Brown, R. G. and Marsden, C. D. (1991), 'Dual task performance and processing in normal subjects and patients with Parkinson's disease', *Brain*, 114A:1, pp. 215–31.

Broyard, Anatole (1992), *Intoxicated by My Illness: And Other Writings on Life and Death* (comp. and ed. A. Broyard), New York: Clarkson N. Potter.

Bruin, Natalie de, Doan, Jon B., Turnbull, George, Suchowersky, Oksana, Bonfield, Stephan, Hu, Bin and Brown, Lesley A. (2010), 'Walking with music is a safe and viable tool for gait training in Parkinson's disease: The effect of a 13 week feasibility study on single and dual task walking', *Parkinson's Disease*, pp. 1–9.

Bunce, Jill (2002), 'The living death: Dance movement therapy with Parkinson's patients', in D. Waller (ed.), *Art Therapies and Progressive Illness: Nameless Dread*, Hove: Brunner-Routledge, pp. 27–46.

Bury, Michael (1997), *Health and Illness in a Changing Society*, London: Routledge.

Butterworth, Jo (2009), 'Too many cooks? A framework for dance making and devising', in J. Butterworth and L. Wildschut (eds), *Choreography in Contexts: A Critical Reader*, London: Routledge, pp. 177–94.

Caines, Rebecca and Heble, Ajay (eds) (2015), *The Improvisation Studies Reader: Spontaneous Acts*, London: Routledge.

Calvo-Merino, Beatriz, Glaser, Daniel E., Grèzes, Julie, Passingham, Richard E. and Haggard, Patrick (2005), 'Action observation and acquired motor skills: An fMRI study with expert dancers', *Cerebral Cortex*, 15:8, pp. 1243–49.

—— (2006), 'Seeing or doing? Influence of visual and motor familiarity in action observation', *Current Biology*, 16, pp. 1905–10.

Calvo-Merino, Beatriz, Jola, Corrine, Glazer, Daniel and Haggard, Patrick (2008), 'Towards a sensori-motor aesthetics of performing art', *Consciousness and Cognition*, 17:3, pp. 911–22.

Carnwath, John D. and Brown, Alan S. (2014), *Understanding the Value and Impacts of Cultural Experiences: A Literature Review*, London: Arts Council England.

Cavarero, Adriana (1997), 'Birth, love and politics', *Radical Philosophy*, 86:Nov/Dec, pp. 19–23.

Channel 4 News (2015), 'How ballet is helping people with Parkinson's find a new lease of life', Facebook, 27 October, https://www.facebook.com/Channel4News/videos/10153301238136 939/?_rdr=p. Accessed 28 October 2015.

Charcot, Jean-Marie (1892), *Oeuvres complètes de J.M. Charcot: Leçons sur les maladies du système nerveux*, vol. 1, Paris: Bourneville.

Clark, David (1973), 'The concept of community: A re-examination', *Sociological Review*, 21, pp. 397–416.

Clift, Stephen, Camic, Paul M., Chapman, Brian, Clayton, Gavin, Daykin, Norma, Eades, Guy, Parkinson, Clive, Secker, Jenny, Stickley, Theo and White, Mike (2009), 'The state of arts and health in England', *Arts & Health: An International Journal for Research, Policy and Practice*, 1:1, pp. 6–35.

Cinconze, Roberto (2015), *Dance for Health Italia: Eva* (trans. A. Trevisan), Bassano del Grappa: Operaestate, https://vimeo.com/123652602. Accessed 3 September 2015.

Cohen, Selma Jeanne (1982), *Next Week Swan Lake: Reflections on Dance and Dances*, Middletown, CT: Wesleyan University Press.

Connatty, John, McKenny, Ellen and Swindlehurst, Kate (2013), 'Tango and Parkinson's: The view from the dance floor', *Animated*, Winter, pp. 16–18.

Connolly, Mary Kate and Redding, Emma (2010), *Dancing Towards Well-Being in the Third Age: Literature Review of the Impact of Dance on Health and Well-Being Among Older People*, London: Trinity Laban Conservatoire of Music and Dance.

Conroy, Collette (2015), 'Editorial: Aesthetics and participation…', *Research in Drama Education: The Journal of Applied Theatre and Performance*, 20:1, pp. 1–11.

Conroy, Renee M. (2013), 'Responding bodily', *Journal of Aesthetics and Art Criticism*, 71:2, pp. 203–10.

Conway, Kathlyn (2007), *Beyond Words: Illness and the Limits of Expression*, Albuquerque, NM: University of New Mexico Press.

Cooper Albright, Ann (1997), *Choreographing Difference: The Body and Identity in Contemporary Dance*, Middletown, CT: Wesleyan University Press.

Corbin, Juliet M. (2003), 'The body in health and illness', *Qualitative Health Research*, 13, pp. 256–67.

Crehan, Kate (2011), *Community Art: An Anthropological Perspective*, London: Berg.

Croft, Clare (2017), *Queer Dance: Meanings and Makings*, New York: Oxford University Press.

Cummings, Jeffrey L. (1992), 'Depression and Parkinson's disease: A review', *American Journal of Psychiatry*, 149, pp. 443–54.

Cushnie, Daphne (2008), 'We're still dancing', *Animated*, Winter, pp. 16–17.

D'Anna, Giulio (2014), *Parkin'Son*, composed by Maarten Bokslag, The Place, London, 24 November.

Dance for PD (2011), *Training Handbook*, New York: Mark Morris Dance Group / Brooklyn Parkinson Group.

—— (2014), 'Training', http://danceforparkinsons.org/training workshops. Accessed 28 November 2014.

—— (2017), 'About Dance for PD', https://danceforparkinsons.org. Accessed 28 October 2017.

Danto, Arthur C. (2003), *The Abuse of Beauty: Aesthetics and the Concept of Art*, Chicago, IL: Open Court.

Davies, David (2013), 'Dancing around the issues: Prospects for an empirically grounded philosophy of dance', *Journal of Aesthetics and Art Criticism*, 71:2, pp. 195–202.

—— (2014), '"This is your brain on art": What can philosophy of art learn from neuroscience', in G. Currie, M. Kieran, A. Meskin and J. Robson (eds), *Aesthetics and the Sciences of Mind*, Oxford: Oxford University Press, pp. 57–74.

Davies, Telroy (2010), 'Mobility: AXIS dancers push the boundaries of access', in B. Henderson and N. Ostrander (eds), *Understanding Disability Studies and Performance Studies*, Abingdon: Routledge, pp. 43–63.

Davis, Jennifer C., Robertson, M. Clare, Ashe, Maureen C., Liu-Ambrose, Teresa, Khan, Karim M. and Marra, Carlo A. (2010), 'International comparison of cost of falls in older adults living in the community: A systematic review', *Osteoporosis International*, 21, pp. 1295–306.

Dawson, Bob (2007), Parkinson's Patients: Yes We Can Dance, http://parkinsonsdance.blogspot.co.uk. Accessed 14 November 2014.

Dean, Cat (2013), 'Dreaming with their feet', *EPDA Plus*, Summer:22, pp. 20–23.

Deane, Katherine H.O., Flaherty, Helen, Daly, David J., Pascoe, Roland, Penhale, Bridget, Clarke, Carl E., Sackley, Catherine and Storey, Stacey (2014), 'Priority setting partnership to identify the top 10 research priorities for the management of Parkinson's disease', *BMJ Open*, 4:12, http://bmjopen.bmj.com/content/4/12/e006434.full. Accessed 17 December 2014.

DeFrantz, Thomas F. (2005), 'African American dance: Philosophy, aesthetics and "beauty"', *Topoi*, 24, pp. 93–102.

Delignières, Didier and Torre, Kjerstin (2009), 'Fractal dynamics of human gait: A reassessment of the 1996 data of Hausdorff et al.', *Journal of Applied Physiology*, 106:4, pp. 1272–79.

Dhami, Prabhjot, Moreno, Sylvain and DeSouza, Joseph (2015), 'New framework for rehabilitation – Fusion of cognitive and physical rehabilitation: The hope for dancing', *Frontiers in Psychology*, https://www.frontiersin.org/articles/10.3389/fpsyg.2014.01478/full. Accessed 10 March 2015.

Dreu, Miek J. de, Kwakkel, Gert and van Wegen, Erwin E. H. (2014), 'Rhythmic auditory stimulation (RAS) in gait rehabilitation for patients with Parkinson's disease: A research perspective', in M. H. Thaut and V. Hoemberg (eds), *Handbook of Neurologic Music Therapy*, Oxford: Oxford University Press, pp. 69–93.

Dreu, Miek J. de, van der Wilk, A. S. Dymphy, Poppe, E., Kwakkel, Gert and van Wegen, Erwin E. H. (2012), 'Rehabilitation, exercise therapy and music in patients with Parkinson's disease: A meta-analysis of the effects of music-based movement therapy on walking ability, balance and quality of life', *Parkinsonism & Related Disorders*, 18, pp. S114–19.

Duff, Joanne, Gillespie, Anna and Fogg, Amanda (2011), 'Making it happen', *Animated*, Autumn, pp. 26–28.

Duffy, Stephen (1993), *The Dynamics of Grace: Perspectives in Theological Anthropology*, Collegeville, MN: The Liturgical Press.

Dujardin, Kathy and Defebvre, Luc (2012), 'Apathy in Parkinson's disease: Clinical features, mechanisms and assessment', *Revue Neurologique*, 168:8&9, pp. 598–604.

Duncan, Ryan P. and Earhart, Gammon M. (2012), 'Randomized controlled trial of community based dancing to modify disease progression in Parkinson disease', *Neurorehabilitation and Neural Repair*, 26:2, pp. 132–43.

Earhart, Gammon (2009), 'Dance as therapy for individuals with Parkinson's disease', *European Journal of Physical Rehabilitative Medicine*, 45:2, pp. 231–38.

Ebersbach, Georg, Ebersbach, Almut, Edler, Daniela, Kaufhold, Olaf, Kusch, Matthias, Kupsch, Andreas and Wissel, Jörg (2010), 'Comparing exercise in Parkinson's disease: The Berlin BIG study', *Movement Disorders*, 25:12, pp. 1902–08.

Eco, Umberto (2004), *On Beauty: A History of a Western Idea* (trans. A. McEwen), London: Secker & Warburg.

Eisenhauer, Jennifer (2007), 'Just looking and staring back: Challenging ableism through disability performance art', *Studies in Art Education*, 49:1, pp. 7–22.

Eliade, Mircea (1959), *The Sacred and the Profane: The Nature of Religion*, New York: Harcourt, Brace and World.

EPDA (European Parkinson's Disease Association) (2011), *Life with Parkinson's*, Brussels: EPDA.
—— (2014), *Move for Change*, London: EPDA, http://www.epda.eu.com/en/projects/move-for-change/. Accessed 24 November 2014.

Eyigor, Sibel, Karapolat, Hale, Durmaz, Berrin, Ibisoglu, Ugur and Cakir, Serap (2009), 'A randomized controlled trial of Turkish Folklore dance on the physical performance, balance, depression and quality of life in older women', *Archives of Gerontology and Geriatrics*, 48:1, pp. 84–88.

Farrell, Lisa, Hollingsworth, Bruce, Propper, Carol and Shields, Michael A. (2014), 'The socioeconomic gradient in physical inactivity: Evidence from one million adults in England', *Social Science and Medicine*, 123, December, pp. 55–63.

Federici, Ario, Bellagamba, Silvia and Rocchi, Marco B. L. (2005), 'Does dance-based training improve balance in adult and young old subjects? A pilot randomized controlled trial', *Aging Clinical and Experimental Research*, 17, pp. 385–89.

Fogg, Amanda (2008), '"We are all dancers": Dance and Parkinson's disease', *Animated*, Spring, http://www.communitydance.org.uk/DB/animated-library/we-are-all-dancersdance andparkinsonsdisease.html?ps=VYt37UqnDCx7swj9dZ5U0nV_lsbQP&lib=14043. Accessed 25 November 2014.

Forsyth, Christopher B., Shannon, Kathleen M., Kordower, Jeffrey H., Voigt, Robin M., Shaikh, Maliha, Jaglin, Jean A., Estes, Jacob D., Dodiya, Hemraj B. and Keshavarzian, Ali (2011), 'Increased intestinal permeability correlates with sigmoid mucosa alpha-synuclein staining and endotoxin exposure markers in early Parkinson's disease', *PLOS One*, http://journals.plos. org/plosone/article?id=10.1371/journal.pone.0028032. Accessed 29 October 2014.

Foster, Erin, Golden, Laura, Duncan, Ryan P. and Earhart, Gammon M. (2013), 'Community-based Argentine tango dance program is associated with increased activity participation among individuals with Parkinson's disease', *Archives of Physical Medicine and Rehabilitation*, 94:2, pp. 240–49.

Foster, Susan Leigh (2011), *Choreographing Empathy: Kinesthesia in Performance*, New York: Routledge.

Fox, Alice and MacPherson, Hannah (2015), *Inclusive Arts Practice and Research: A Critical Manifesto*, London: Routledge.

Fraleigh, Sondra Horton (1987), *Dance and the Lived Body: A Descriptive Aesthetics*, Pittsburgh: University of Pittsburgh Press.

Frank, Arthur (1991), 'For a sociology of the body: An analytical review', in M. Featherstone, M. Hepworth and B. Turner (eds), *The Body: Social Process and Cultural Theory*, London: Sage, pp. 36–102.

—— (2010), *Letting Stories Breathe: A Socio-Narratology*, Chicago, IL: University of Chicago Press.

—— ([1995] 2013), *The Wounded Storyteller: Body, Illness and Ethics*, Chicago, IL: University of Chicago Press.

Freire, Paulo (1993), *Pedagogy of the Oppressed* (trans. M. Bergman Ramos), London: Penguin Books.

Gallese, Vittorio and Goldman, Alvin (1998), 'Mirror neurons and the simulation theory of mind-reading', *Trends in Cognitive Science*, 2:12, pp. 493–501.

Gao, Qiang, Leung, Aaron, Yonghong, Yang, Wei, Qingchuan, Guan, Min, Jia, Chenseng and He, Chengqi (2014), 'Effects of Tai Chi on balance and fall prevention in Parkinson's disease: A randomized controlled trial', *Clinical Rehabilitation*, 28:8, pp. 748–53.

Garland-Thompson, Rosemarie (2002), 'Integrating disability, transforming feminist theory', *NWSA Journal*, 14:3, pp. 1–32.

Giling, Martin W. L. (2014), 'When I dance I feel like a different man', *Dans MAGAZINE*, 6, pp. 36–39.

Gillette, Monica (2015), Physical Thinking, 11 August, https://hafraah.wordpress.com/2015/08/ 11/physical-thinking/. Accessed 13 August 2015.

Goering, Sara (2002), 'Beyond the medical model? Disability, formal justice and the exception for the profoundly impaired', *Kennedy Institute of Ethics Journal*, 12:4, pp. 373–88.

Goldman, Danielle (2010), *I Want to Be Ready: Improvised Dance as a Practice of Freedom*, Ann Arbor, MI: University of Michigan Press.

Gombrich, Ernst H. (1945), 'Botticelli's mythologies: A study in the neoplatonic symbolism of his circle', *Journal of the Warburg and Courtauld Institutes*, 8, pp. 7–60.

Grace, Alicia (2009), 'Dancing with lassitude: A dramaturgy from limbo', *Research in Drama Education: The Journal of Applied Theatre and Performance*, 14:1, pp. 15–29.

Green, Jill (2000), 'Power, service and reflexivity in a community dance project', *Research in Dance Education*, 1:1, pp. 53–67.

Grenier, Amanda and Phillipson, Chris (2014), 'Rethinking agency in late life: Structural and interpretative approaches', in J. Baars, J. Dohmen, A. Grenier and C. Phillipson (eds), *Ageing, Meaning and Social Structure*, Bristol: Policy Press, pp. 55–79.

Gubrium, Jaber F. and Holstein, James (1995), 'Individual agency, the ordinary and postmodern life', *The Sociological Quarterly*, 36:3, pp. 555–70.

Gumber, Anil, Ramaswamy, Bhanu, Ibbotson, Rachel, Ismail, Mubarak, Thongchundee, Oranuch, Harrop, Deborah, Allmark, Peter and Rauf, Abdur (2017), *Economic, Social and Financial Cost of Parkinson's on Individuals, Carers and Families in the UK*, Sheffield: Sheffield Hallam University, https://www.shu.ac.uk/research/specialisms/centre-for-health-and-social care-research/reports/economic-social-and-financial-cost-of-parkinsons-on individuals-carers-and-their-families. Accessed 15 September 2017.

Hackney, Madeleine E. and Bennett, Crystal G. (2014), 'Dance therapy for individuals with Parkinson's disease: Improving quality of life', *Journal of Parkinsonism and Restless Legs Syndrome*, 4, pp. 17–25.

Hackney, Madeleine E. and Earhart, Gammon M. (2009), 'Effects of dance on movement control in Parkinson's disease: A comparison of Argentine tango and American ballroom', *Journal of Rehabilitative Medicine*, 41, pp. 475–81.

—— (2010), 'Effects of dance on gait and balance in Parkinson's disease: A comparison of partnered and nonpartnered dance movement', *Neurorehabilitation and Neural Repair*, 24, pp. 384–92.

Hackney, Madeleine E., Kantorovich, Svetlana and Earhart, Gammon M. (2007), 'A study on the effects of Argentine tango as a form of partnered dance for those with Parkinson disease and the healthy elderly', *American Journal of Dance Therapy*, 29, pp. 109–27.

Hall, Kirk (2015), Shaky Paws Grampa, http://www.shakypawsgrampa.com. Accessed 1 April 2015.

Hamera, Judith (2007), *Dancing Communities: Performance, Difference and Connection in the Global City*, Basingstoke: Palgrave Macmillan.

Hanna, Judith Lynne (2015), *Dancing to Learn: The Brain's Cognition, Emotion and Movement*, Lanham, MD: Rowman and Littlefield.

Hausdorff, Jeffrey M. (2009), 'Gait dynamics in Parkinson's disease: Common and distinct behavior among stride length, gait variability and fractal-like scaling', *Chaos: An Interdisciplinary Journal of Nonlinear Science*, 19:2, http://scitation.aip.org/content/aip/journal/chaos/19/2/10.1063/1.3147408. Accessed 5 January 2015.

Hausdorff, Jeffrey M., Lowenthal, Justine, Herman, Talia, Gruendlinger, Leor, Peretz, Chava and Giladi, Nir (2007), 'Rhythmic auditory stimulation modulates gait variability in Parkinson's disease', *European Journal of Neuroscience*, 26:8, pp. 2045–53.

Hausdorff, Jeffrey M., Purdon, Patrick L., Peng, Chung-Kang., Ladin, Zvi, Wei, Jeanne Y. and Golderger, Ary R. (1996), 'Fractal dynamics of human gait: Stability of long-range correlations in stride interval fluctuation', *Journal of Applied Physiology*, 80:5, pp. 1448–57.

Heiberger, Lisa, Maurer, Christoph, Amtage, Florian, Mendez-Balbuena, Ignacio, Schulte-Mönting, Jürgen, Hepp Reymond, Marie-Claude and Kristeva, Rumyana (2011), 'Impact of a weekly dance class on the functional mobility and on the quality of life of individuals with Parkinson's disease', *Frontiers in Aging Neuroscience*, 3:14, pp. 1–15.

Henderson, Bruce and Ostrander, Noam (2010), *Understanding Disability Studies and Performance Studies*, Abingdon: Routledge.

Hennion, Antoine and Grenier, Line (2000), 'Sociology of art: New stakes in a post critical time', in S. R. Quah and A. Sales (eds), *International Handbook of Sociology*, London: Sage, pp. 341–45.

Higgins, Kathleen Marie (1996), 'Whatever happened to beauty? A response to Danto', *Journal of Aesthetics and Art Criticism*, 54:3, pp. 281–84.

Hill, Richard (2009), 'An afternoon with Prof J Eric Ahlskog', *SPRING Times: Research and Action to Cure Parkinson's*, 53, pp. 4–7.

Hirsch, Mark A., Hammond, Flora and Hirsch, Helmut V. B. (2008), 'From research to practice: Rehabilitation of persons living with Parkinson's disease', *Topics in Geriatric Rehabilitation*, 24:2, pp. 92–98.

Hoehn, Margaret M. and Yahr, Melvin D. (1967), 'Parkinsonism: Onset, progression, and mortality', *Neurology*, 17, pp. 427–42.

Hogarth, William (1753), *The Analysis of Beauty*, London: J. Reeves.

Holden, John (2004), 'Capturing cultural value: How culture has become a tool in government policy', *Demos*, https://www.demos.co.uk/files/CapturingCulturalValue.pdf?1240939425. Accessed 15 November 2013.

Houston, Sara (2011), 'The methodological challenges of research into dance for people with Parkinson's', *Dance Research*, 29, pp. 327–49.

—— (2014), 'Moved to dance: Socially engaged dance facilitation', in M. E. Anderson and D. Risner (eds), *Hybrid Lives of Teaching Artists in Dance and Theatre Arts: A Critical Reader*, New York: Cambria Press, pp. 133–54.

—— (2015), 'Feeling lovely: An examination of the value of beauty for people dancing with Parkinson's', *Dance Research Journal*, 47:1, pp. 26–43.

Houston, Sara and McGill, Ashley (2011), *English National Ballet Dance for Parkinson's: An Investigative Study*, research report 1, London: University of Roehampton.

—— (2013), 'A mixed-methods study into ballet for people living with Parkinson's', *Arts & Health: An International Journal for Research, Policy and Practice*, 5:2, pp. 103–19.

—— (2015), *English National Ballet Dance for Parkinson's: An Investigative Study 2, A Report on a Three Year Mixed-Methods Research Study*, research report 2, London: English National Ballet.

Hove, Michael J., Suzuki, Kazuki, Uchitomi, Hirotaka, Orimo, Satoshi and Miyake, Yoshihiro (2012), 'Interactive rhythmic auditory stimulation reinstates natural 1/$f$ structure in gait of Parkinson's patients', *PLOS ONE*, http://www.plosone.org/article/info%3Adoi%2F10.1371%2Fjournal.pone.003 600#pone-0032600-g003. Accessed 23 December 2014.

Howe, Tracey E., Lövgreen, Brenda, Cody, Frederick W. J., Ashton, Vicki J. and Oldham, Jacqueline A. (2003), 'Auditory cues can modify the gait of persons with early-stage Parkinson's disease: A method for enhancing Parkinsonian walking performance?' *Clinical Rehabilitation*, 17:4, pp. 363–67.

HSCIC (Health and Social Care Information Centre) (2012), *Health Survey for England*, Health and Social Care Information Centre, http://www.hscic.gov.uk/catalogue/PUB13218/ HSE2012-Ch2-Phys-act adults.pdf. Accessed 15 December 2014.

Hughes, Bill and Paterson, Kevin (1997), 'The social model of disability and the disappearing body: Towards a sociology of impairment', *Disability and Society*, 12:3, pp. 325–40.

Hui, Elsie, Chui, Bo Tsan-Keung and Woo, Jean (2009), 'Effects of dance on physical and psychological well-being in older persons', *Archives in Gerontology and Geriatrics*, 49:1, pp. e45–50.

Hybbinette, Pelle (2017), *Moving Skåne*, Malmö: Skånes Dansteater.

Inzelberg, Rivka (2013), 'The awakening of artistic creativity and Parkinson's disease', *Behavioural Science*, 127:2, pp. 256–61.

Iverson, Dave (2014a), *Capturing Grace*, USA: Kikim Media LLC.

——— (2014b), 'About the film', http://www.capturinggracefilm.com/what-we-do/. Accessed 17 February 2015.

Jacobs, Jesse V. and Horack, Fay B. (2006), 'Abnormal proprioceptive-motor integration contributes to hypometric postural responses of subjects with Parkinson's disease', *Neuroscience*, 141:2, pp. 999–1009.

Jancovich, Leila (2015), 'The participation myth', *International Journal of Cultural Policy*, 23:1, http://www.tandfonline.com/doi/abs/10.1080/10286632.2015.1027698. Accessed 18 March 2016.

Jasper, Linda (1995), 'Tensions in the definition of community dance', *Border Tensions: Dance and Discourse – Proceedings from the Fifth Study of Dance Conference*, 20–23 April, Guildford: University of Surrey, pp. 181–90.

Jeffery, Erica Rose (2014a), *Dance for Parkinson's Pilot Research: Short Report*, Brisbane: Queensland Ballet.

——— (2014b), 'Dance for Parkinson's in Australia: A journey of movement and music – Building confidence, creativity and community', Ausdance, http://ausdance.org.au/articles/details/dance-for parkinsons-in-australia. Accessed 7 March 2016.

Jenkinson, Crispin, Fitzpatrick, Ray, Peto, Viv, Greenhall, Richard and Hyman, Nigel (1997), 'The Parkinson's disease questionnaire (PDQ-39): Development and validation of a Parkinson's disease summary index score', *Age and Ageing*, 26, pp. 353–57.

Joutsa, Juho, Martikainen, Kirsti and Kaasinen, Valtteri (2012), 'Parallel appearance of compulsive behaviours and artistic creativity in Parkinson's disease', *Case Reports in Neurology*, 4, pp. 77–83.

Jurecic, Ann (2012), *Illness as Narrative*, Pittsburgh, PA: University of Pittsburgh Press.

Kelly, Owen (1984), *Community, Art and the State: Storming the Citadels*, London: Comedia.

Kelsall, Kate (2014), Shake, Rattle and Roll: An Insider's View of Parkinson's Disease and DBS, http://katekelsall.typepad.com/my_weblog/parkinsons-dance/. Accessed 24 November 2014.

Keogh, Justin W. L., Kilding, Andrew, Pidgeon, Phillippa, Ashley, Linda and Gillis, Dawn (2009), 'Physical benefits of dancing for healthy older adults: A review', *Journal of Aging and Physical Activity*, 17, pp. 479–500.

Klausmann, Anne (2015), 'Treasure chest: My body moves me' (trans. I. Schröder), 3 June, https://hafraah.wordpress.com/2015/06/03/treasure-chest/. Accessed 8 June 2014.

Kostoula, Christina (2012), 'Inclusive dance practice: Barriers to learning', in L. Sanders (ed.), *Dance Teaching and Learning: Shaping Practice*, London: Youth Dance England, pp. 75–82.

Krischer, Sandra (2016), Twitchy Woman: My Adventures with Parkinson's Disease, http://www. twitchywoman.com. Accessed 6 July 2016.

Kulisevsky, Jaime, Pagonabarraga, Javier and Martinez-Corral, Mercè (2009), 'Changes in artistic style and behaviour in Parkinson's disease: Dopamine and creativity', *Journal of Neurology*, 256, pp. 816–19.

Kuppers, Petra (2011), *Disability Culture and Community Performance: Find a Strange and Twisted Shape*, Basingstoke: Palgrave Macmillan.

Lamont, Robyn, Jeffrey, Erica Rose, Moyle, Gene Margaret, Kerr, Graham K. and Brauer, Sandra G. (2016), 'The impact of a six-month dance for Parkinson's program on physical function and wellbeing: A mixed-methods pilot study', *4th World Parkinson Congress,* 20–23 September, Portland, Orgeon.

Leighton, Fran (2009), 'Accountability: The ethics of devising a practice-as-research performance with learning-disabled practitioners', *Research in Drama Education: The Journal of Applied Theatre and Performance*, 14:1, pp. 97–113.

Levin, David Michael (1983), 'Balanchine's formalism', in R. Copeland and M. Cohen (eds), *What is Dance?*, New York: Oxford University Press, pp. 123–45.

Litvan, Irene, Aarsland, Dag, Adler, Charles H., Goldman, Jennifer G., Kulisevsky, Jamie, Mollenhauer, Brit, Rodriguez-Oroz, Maria C., Tröster, Alexander I. and Weintraub, Daniel (2011), 'MDS task force on mild cognitive impairment in Parkinson's disease: Critical review of PD-MCI', *Movement Disorders*, 26:10, pp. 1814–24.

Livia, Anna and Hall, Kira (1997), *Queerly Phrased: Language, Gender and Sexuality*, New York: Oxford University Press.

Lomas, Christine M. (1998), 'Art and the community: Breaking the aesthetic of disempowerment', in S. B. Shapiro (ed.), *Dance, Power, and Difference: Critical and Feminist Perspectives on Dance Education*, Champaign, IL: Human Kinetics, pp. 149–70.

Lutes, Clint (2015), 'Improvisation score', Theatre Freiburg, 19 December.

Machielse, Anja and Hortulanus, Roelof (2014), 'Social ability or social frailty? The balance between autonomy and connectedness in the lives of older people', in J. Baars, J. Dohmen, A. Grenier and C. Phillipson (eds), *Ageing, Meaning and Social Structure*, Bristol: Policy Press.

Mackintosh, Iain (1993), *Architecture, Actor and Audience*, London: Routledge.

Macnaughton, Jane, White, Mike and Stacy, Rosie (2005), 'Researching the benefits of arts in health', *Health Education*, 105:5, pp. 332–39.

Manning, Erin (2009), *Relationscapes: Movement, Art, Philosophy*, Cambridge, MA: MIT Press.

Marchant, David., Sylvester, Jennifer L. and Earhart, Gammon M. (2010), 'Effects of a short duration, high dose contact improvisation dance workshop on parkinson disease: A pilot study', *Complementary Therapies in Medicine*, 18:5, pp. 184–90.

Massumi, Brian (2015), *Politics of Affect*, Cambridge, MA: Polity Press.

McFee, Graham (1992), *Understanding Dance*, London: Routledge.

McGill, Ashley, Houston, Sara and Lee, Raymond (2015), 'Dance for Parkinson's: A new framework for research on its physical, mental, emotional and social benefits', *Complementary Therapies in Medicine*, 22:3, pp. 426–32.

—— (2018), 'Effects of a ballet-based dance intervention on gait variability and balance confidence of people with Parkinson's', *Arts & Health: An International Journal of Research, Policy and Practice*, 11:2, https://www.tandfonline.com/doi/full/10.1080/17533015.2018.1443947. Accessed 14 March 2018.

McIntosh, Gerald C., Brown, Susan H., Rice, Ruth R. and Thaut, Michael H. (1997), 'Rhythmic auditory-motor facilitation of gait patterns in patients with Parkinson's disease', *Journal of Neurology, Neurosurgery & Psychiatry*, 62, pp. 22–26.

McKee, Kathleen E. and Hackney, Madeleine E. (2013), 'The effects of adapted tango on spatial cognition and disease severity in Parkinson's disease', *Journal of Motor Behavior*, 45:6, pp. 519–29.

Menegon, Alessandra, Board, Philip G., Blackburn, Anneke C., Mellick, George D. and Le Couteur, David G. (1998), 'Parkinson's disease, pesticides and glutathoine transferase polymorphisms', *The Lancet*, 352:9137, pp. 1344–46.

Michael J. Fox Foundation (2015), https://www.michaeljfox.org. Accessed 27 January 2014.

Miller, William Ian (1997), *The Anatomy of Disgust*, Cambridge, MA: Harvard University Press.

Miller, William L. and Crabtree, Benjamin F. (2000), 'Clinical research', in N. K. Denzin and Y. S. Lincoln (eds), *Handbook of Qualitative Research*, 2nd ed., Thousand Oaks, CA: Sage, pp. 607–31.

Monk, Samuel H. (1944), 'A grace beyond the reach of art', *Journal of the History of Ideas*, 5:2, pp. 131–50.

Montero, Barbara (2006), 'Proprioceiving someone else's movement', *Philosophical Explorations*, 9:2, pp. 149–61.

—— (2016), *Thought in Action: Expertise and the Conscious Mind*, Oxford: Oxford University Press.

Morris, Gay (2009), 'Dance studies/cultural studies', *Dance Research Journal*, 41:1, pp. 82–100, http://muse.jhu.edu/journals/dance_research_journal/v041/41.1.morris.html. Accessed 4 August 2010.

Murcia, Cynthia Quiroga, Kreutz, Gunter, Clift, Stephen and Bongard, Stephan (2010), 'Shall we dance? An exploration of the perceived benefits of dancing on well-being', *Arts & Health: An International Journal for Research, Policy and Practice*, 2:2, pp. 149–63.

Nevile, Jennifer (1991), '"Certain sweet movements": The development of the concept of grace in 15th-century Italian dance and painting', *Dance Research*, 9:1, pp. 3–12.

Niaah, Sonjah Stanley (2010), *DanceHall: From Slave Ship to Ghetto*, Ottawa: University of Ottawa Press.

Nieuwboer, Alice (2009), 'Exercise for Parkinson's disease: The evidence under scrutiny', *Developing the Disease Modifying Possibilities of Exercise on Parkinson's: Special Parkinson's Research Interest Group of the Parkinson's Disease Society Conference*, Gatwick, 24–25 September.

Nijhof, Gerhard (1995), 'Parkinson's disease as a problem of shame in public appearance', *Sociology of Health & Illness*, 17:2, pp. 193–205.

Nijkrake, Maarten, Keus, Samyra, Overeem, Sebastiaan, Oostendorp, Rob, Vliet Vlieland, Thea, Mulleners, Wim, Hoogervaard, Edo, Bloem, Bas and Munneke, Marten (2010), 'The ParkinsonNet concept: Development, implementation and initial experience', *Movement Disorders*, 25:7, pp. 823–29.

Noland, Carrie (2009), *Agency and Embodiment: Performing Gestures/Producing Culture*, Cambridge, MA: Harvard University Press.

Novack, Cynthia J. (1993), 'Ballet, gender and cultural power', in H. Thomas (ed.), *Dance, Gender and Culture*, Basingstoke: Palgrave Macmillan, pp. 34–48.

Nussbaum, Martha C. (2007), *Frontiers of Justice: Disability, Nationality, Species Membership*, Cambridge, MA: The Belknap Press of Harvard University Press.

—— (2011), *Creating Capabilities: The Human Development Approach*, Cambridge, MA: The Belknap Press of Harvard University Press.

O'Connor, Barbara (1997), 'Safe sets: Women, dance and "communitas"', in H. Thomas (ed.), *Dance in the City*, Basingstoke: Macmillan, pp. 149–72.

Oliver, Michael (1990), *The Politics of Disablement*, London: Macmillan.

Olsson, Malin, Stafström, Lena and Söderberg, Siv (2013), 'Meanings of fatigue for women with Parkinson's disease', *Qualitative Health Research*, 23:6, pp. 741–48.

Oman, John (1919), *Grace and Personality*, Cambridge: Cambridge University Press.

Pacchetti, Claudio, Francesca Mancini, Roberto Aglieri, Cira Fundaro, Emila Martignoni and Giuseppe Nappi (2000), 'Active music therapy in Parkinson's disease: An integrative method for motor and emotional rehabilitation', *Psychosomatic Medicine*, 62, pp. 386–93.

Pakes, Anna (2006), 'Dance's mind-body problem', *Dance Research*, 24:2, pp. 87–104.

Palfreman, Jon (2015), *Brain Storms: The Race to Unlock the Mysteries of Parkinson's*, London: Rider.

Parkinson, James (1817), *An Essay on the Shaking Palsy*, London: Sherwood, Neely and Jones.

Parkinson's UK (2013), 'What is Parkinson's?', http://www.parkinsons.org.uk/about_parkinsons/what_is_parkinsons.aspx. Accessed 3 February 2013.

—— (2014), 'About Parkinson's', http://www.parkinsons.org.uk/content/about-parkinsons. Accessed 18 November 2014.

Paul, Ray (2009), *Living with Parkinson's Disease: Shake Rattle and Roll*, London: RAIL.

People Dancing (2015), *Annual Report 2014–2015*, Leicester: People Dancing, The Foundation for Community Dance.

Petzinger, Giselle M., Fisher, Beth E., McEwen, Sarah, Walsh, John P. and Jakowec, Michael W. (2013), 'Exercise-enhanced neuroplasticity targeting motor and cognitive circuitry in Parkinson's disease', *The Lancet Neurology*, 12, pp. 716–26.

Platz, Thomas, Brown, Richard G. and Marsden, C. David (1998), 'Training improves the speed of aimed movements in Parkinson's disease', *Brain*, 121, pp. 505–14.

Potts, John (2009), *A History of Charisma*, Basingstoke: Palgrave Macmillan.

Price, Jonathan (2015), 'Contesting agendas of participation in the arts', *Journal of Arts & Communities*, 7:1&2, pp. 17–31.

Public Health England (2014), *Everybody Active, Everyday: What Works: The Evidence*, London: PHE publications.

Quinn, Pamela (2013), 'Dancing with outliers: Let's study the best-case scenarios in managing Parkinson's disease', *Neurology Now*, April/May, p. 40.

RAM publications (2016), 'Art backlist', http://www.rampub.com/art/backlist6. Accessed 13 July 2016.

Ran, Faye (2007), 'Modern tragicomedy and the fool', in D. Robb (ed.), *Clowns, Fools and Picaros: Popular Forms in Theatre, Fiction and Film*, Amsterdam: Rodopi, pp. 25–36.

Rehfeld, Kathrin, Müller, Patrick, Aye, Norman, Schmicker, Marlen, Dordevic, Milos, Kaufmann, Jörn, Hökelmann, Anita and Müller, Notger G. (2017), 'Dancing or fitness sport? The effects of two training programs on hippocampal plasticity and balance ability in healthy seniors', *Frontiers in Human Neuroscience*, 11:305, http://journal.frontiersin.org/article/10.3389/fnhum.2017.00305/full. Accessed 30 August 2017.

Reynolds, Dee (2012), 'Kinesthetic empathy and the dance's body: From emotion to affect', in D. Reynolds and M. Reason (eds), *Kinesthetic Empathy in Creative and Cultural Practices*, Bristol: Intellect, pp. 121–36.

Reynolds, Dee and Reason, Matthew (eds) (2012), *Kinesthetic Empathy in Creative and Cultural Practices*, Bristol: Intellect.

Ricoeur, Paul (2007), *Freedom and Nature: The Voluntary and the Involuntary* (trans. E. V. Kohák), Evanston, IL: Northwestern University Press.

Riddoch, Chris, Puig-Ribera, Anna and Cooper, Ashley (1998), *Effectiveness of Physical Activity Promotion Schemes in Primary Care: A Review*, London: Health Education Authority.

Rizzolatti, Giacomo, Fadiga, Luciano, Gallese, Vittorio and Fogassi, Leonardo (1996), 'Premotor cortex and the recognition of motor actions', *Cognitive Brain Research*, 3:2, pp. 131–41.

Roehampton Dance (2010), 'Researching Dance for Parkinson's', http://roehamptondance.com/parkinsons. Accessed 20 December 2010.

Sacks, Oliver ([1973] 1990), *Awakenings*, London: Picador.

—— (2007), *Musicophilia: Tales of Music and the Brain*, London: Picador.

Sandahl, Carrie and Auslander, Phillip (eds) (2005), *Bodies in Commotion: Disability and Performance*, Ann Arbor, MI: The University of Michigan Press.

Scarborough, Peter, Bhatnager, Prache, Wickramasinghe, Kremlin K., Allender, Steve, Foster, Charlie and Rayner, Mike (2011), 'The economic burden of ill health due to diet, physical inactivity, smoking, alcohol and obesity in the UK: An update to 2006–07 NHS costs', *Journal of Public Health*, 33:4, pp. 527–35.

Scarry, Elaine (2000), *On Beauty and Being Just*, London: Duckworth Overlook.

Schapira, Tony (2008), *Understanding Parkinson's Disease*, Poole: Family Doctor Books.

Scheperjans, Filip, Aho, Velma, Pereira, Pedro A.B., Koskinen, Kaisa, Pekkonen, Eero, Haapaniemi, Elena, Kaakkola, Seppo, Eerola-Rautio, Johanna, Pohja, Marjatta, Kinnunen, Esko, Murros, Kari and Auvinen, Petri (2014), 'Gut microbiota are related to Parkinson's disease and clinical phenotype', *Movement Disorders*, 30:3, pp. 350–58.

Schulman, Lisa M., Taback, Robin L., Rabinstein, A. A. and Weiner, William J. (2002), 'Non recognition of depression and other non-motor symptoms in Parkinson's disease', *Parkinsonism and Related Disorders*, 8:3, pp. 193–97.

Sennett, Richard (2003), *Respect: The Formation of Character in an Age of Inequality*, London: Penguin Books.

Shanahan, Joanne, Morris, Meg E., Bhriain, Orfhlaith N., Saunders, Jean-Ann and Clifford, Amanda M. (2015), 'Dance for people with Parkinson disease: What is the evidence telling us?', *Archives of Physical Medicine and Rehabilitation*, 96:1, pp. 141–53.

Shanahan, Joanne, Morris, Meg E., Bhriain, Orfhlaith N., Volpe, Daniele, Richardson, Margaret and Clifford, Amanda M. (2015), 'Is Irish set dancing feasible for people with Parkinson's disease in Ireland?', *Complementary Therapies in Clinical Practice*, 21:1, pp. 47–51.

Sheets-Johnstone, Maxine ([1966] 1979), *The Phenomenology of Dance*, London: Dance Books.

—— (1999), 'Emotion and movement: A beginning empirical phenomenological analysis of their relationship', *Journal of Consciousness Studies*, 6:11–12, pp. 259–77.

—— ([1999] 2011), *The Primacy of Movement*, Philadelphia: John Benjamins.

Silvers, Anita (2002), 'The crooked timber of humanity: Disability, ideology and the aesthetic', in M. Corker and T. Shakespeare (eds), *Disability/Postmodernity: Embodying Disability Theory*, London: Continuum, pp. 228–42.

Skelton, D., Young, A., Walker, A. and Hoinville, E. (1999), *Physical Activity in Later Life: Further Analysis of the Allied Dunbar National Fitness Survey and the Health Education Authority National Survey of Activity and Health*, London: Health Education Authority.

Snare, Gerald (1971), 'Spencer's fourth grace', *Journal of the Warburg and Courtauld Institutes*, 34, pp. 350–55.

Snijders, Anke H. and Bloem, Bastiaan R. (2010), 'Cycling for freezing of gait', *The New England Journal of Medicine*, 362:e46, http://www.nejm.org/doi/full/10.1056/NEJMicm0810287#t=article. Accessed 20 October 2017.

Solimeo, Samantha (2009), *With Shaking Hands: Aging with Parkinson's Disease in America's Heartland*, New Brunswick: Rutgers University Press.

Soliveri, Paola, Brown, Richard G., Jahanshahi, Marjan and Marsden, C. David (1992), 'Effect of practice on performance of a skilled motor task in patients with Parkinson's disease', *Journal of Neurology, Neurosurgery and Psychiatry*, 55:6, pp. 454–60.

Soriano, Christina T. and Batson, Glenna (2011), 'Dance-making with adults with Parkinson's disease: One teacher's process of constructing a modern dance class', *Research in Dance Education*, 12:3, pp. 323–37.

Sparshott, Francis (1995), *A Measured Pace: Towards a Philosophical Understanding of the Arts of Dance*, Toronto: University of Toronto Press.

—— (2004), 'The philosophy of dance: Bodies in motion, bodies at rest', in P. Kivy (ed.), *The Blackwell Guide to Aesthetics*, Oxford: Blackwell Publishing, pp. 276–90.

Spencer, Herbert (1891), *Essays: Scientific, Political and Speculative*, vol. 2, London: Williams and Northgate.

Spink, Erik and Kim, Soo Hyung (n.d.), *Class*, https://pdmovementlab.com/exercise-class/. Accessed 31 October 2017.

Spink, Erik, Joshi, Amitabh Raj and Kraus, Lauren (2013), *With Grace*, https://pdmovementlab.com/art/. Accessed 31 October 2017.

Stoltzfus, Michael J. and Schumm, Darla Y. (2011), 'Beyond models: Some tentative Daoist contributions to disability studies', *Disability Studies Quarterly*, 31:1, http://dsq-sds.org/article/view/1366/1538. Accessed 5 November 2013.

Swain, John and French, Sally (2000), 'Towards an affirmation model of disability', *Disability and Society*, 15:4, pp. 569–82.

Thaut, Michael H., Rathbun, Jennifer A. and Miller, Robert A. (1997), 'Music versus metronome timekeeper in a rhythmic motor task', *International Journal of Arts Medicine*, 5, pp. 4–12.

Thomas, Carol (2007), *Sociologies of Disability and Illness*, Basingstoke: Palgrave Macmillan.

Thomas, Helen (2003), *The Body, Dance and Cultural Theory*, Basingstoke: Palgrave Macmillan.

Thompson, James (2009), *Performance Affects: Applied Theatre and the End of Effect*, Basingstoke: Palgrave Macmillan.

Thomson, Chris (1994), 'Dance and the concept of community', *Focus on Community Dance, Dance and the Child International Journal*, 3, pp. 20–30.

Thornton, Sam (1971), *A Movement Perspective of Rudolf Laban*, London: MacDonald & Evans.

Thurston, Miranda and Green, Ken (2004), 'Adherence to exercise in later life: How can exercise on prescription programmes be made more effective?', *Health Promotion International*, 19:3, pp. 379–87.

Thyreen-Mizingou, Jeannine (2000), 'Grace and ethics in contemporary American poetry: Resituating the other, the world and the self', *Religion & Literature*, 32:1, pp. 67–97.

Tobey, Charlie (2016), 'Class 1 testimonial', http://pamelaquinn.net/class-1/. Accessed 28 December 2016.

Todes, Cecil (1990), *Shadow Over My Brain: A Battle Against Parkinson's Disease*, Gloucestershire: The Windrush Press.

Turner, Bryan S. (1992), *Regulating Bodies: Essays in Medical Sociology*, London: Routledge.

Van der Marck, Marjolein A., Kalf, Johanna G., Sturkenboom, Ingrid H.W.M., Nijkrake, Maarten J., Munneke, Marten and Bloem, Bas R. (2009), 'Multidisciplinary care for patients with Parkinson's disease', *Parkinsonism and Related Disorders*, 1553, pp. S219–23.

Vasari, Georgio ([1550] 1991), *The Lives of the Artists* (trans. J. Conaway Bondanella and P. Bondanella), Oxford: Oxford University Press.

Vicary, Staci, Sperling, Matthias, von Zimmermann, Jorina, Richardson, Daniel C. and Orgs, Guido (2017), 'Joint action aesthetics', *PLOS One*, https://doi.org/10.1371/journal.pone.0180101. Accessed 25 October 2017.

Volpe, Daniele, Signorini, Matteo, Marchetto, Anna, Lynch, Timothy and Morris, Meg A. (2013), 'A comparison of Irish set dancing and exercises for people with Parkinson's disease: A phase II feasibility study', *BMC Geriatrics*, 13:54, https://bmcgeriatr.biomedcentral.com/articles/10.1186/1471-2318 13-54. Accessed 4 July 2013.

Warburton, Daniel, Nicol, Crystal Whitney and Bredin, Shannon S. D. (2006), 'Health benefits of physical activity: The evidence', *Canadian Medical Association Journal*, 174:6, pp. 801–09.

Westbrook, Beth K. and McKibben, Helen (1989), 'Dance/movement therapy with groups of outpatients with Parkinson's disease', *American Journal of Dance Therapy*, 11, pp. 27–38.

Westfall, C.W. (2010), 'Classicism and language in architecture', *American Arts Quarterly*, 27:1, http://www.nccsc.net/essays/classicism-and language-architecture. Accessed 18 September 2017.

Westheimer, Olie (2008), 'Why dance for Parkinson's disease?', *Topics in Geriatric Rehabilitation*, 24, pp. 127–40.

Westheimer, Olie, Mcrae, Cynthia, Henchcliffe, Claire, Fesharaki, Arman, Glazman, Sofya, Ene, Heather and Bodis-Wollner, Ivan (2015), 'Dance for PD: A preliminary investigation of effects on motor function and quality of life among persons with Parkinson's disease (PD)', *Journal of Neural Transmission*, 122:9, pp. 1263–70.

White, Mike (2009), *Arts Development in Community Health: A Social Tonic*, Oxford: Radcliffe Publishing.

Wilcock, Ann A. and Hocking, Clare ([1998] 2015), *An Occupational Perspective of Health*, Thorofare, NJ: SLACK Incorporated.

Winston, Joe (2007), 'By way of an introduction, some initial reflections on beauty', *Research in Drama Education: The Journal of Applied Theatre and Performance*, 11:1, pp. 43–45.

Wolff, Janet (1997), 'Reinstating corporeality: Feminisim and body politics', in J. Desmond (ed.), *Meaning in Motion*, Durham, NC and London: Duke University Press, pp. 81–99.

——— (2006), 'Groundless beauty: Feminisim and the aesthetics of uncertainty', *Feminist Theory*, 7:2, pp. 143–58.

Woolhouse, Matthew, Tidhar, Dan and Cross, Ian (2016), 'Effects of interpersonal memory of dancing in time with others', *Frontiers in Psychology*, https://www.frontiersin.org/articles/10.3389/fpsyg.2016.00167/full. Accessed 29 October 2017.

Woolhouse, Matthew, Williams, Stephanie, Shuying, Zheng and General, Ashley (2015), 'Creating dance activities for people with Parkinson's using motion sensor cameras', *International Journal of Health, Wellness and Society*, 5:4, pp. 107–21.

WHO (World Health Organization) (2002), *Towards a Common Language for Functioning, Disability and Health*, Geneva: WHO.

——— (2007), *Steps to Health: A European Framework to Promote Physical Activity for Health*, Denmark: WHO Regional Office for Europe.

World Parkinson Coalition (2016), 'Top 12 videos', http://www.wpc2016.org/page/top12. Accessed 25 September 2016.

Wu, Tao and Hallett, Mark (2005), 'A functional MRI study of automatic movements in patients with Parkinson's disease', *Brain*, 128, pp. 2250–59.

## Dance works (specific performances seen are referenced above)

Bausch, Pina (1975), *The Rite of Spring*, composed by Igor Stravinsky, Tanztheater Wuppertal, Opera House Wuppertal.

D'Anna, Giulio (2011), *Parkin'Son*, composed by Maarten Bokslag, Giulio D'Anna, Rome, Roma Equilibrio.

Deane, Derek (1997) (Marius Petipa and Lev Ivanov [1985]), *Swan Lake*, composed by Peter Ilich Tchaikovsky, English National Ballet, London, Royal Albert Hall.

Eagling, Wayne (2010) (Marius Pepita [1985]), *The Nutcracker*, composed by Peter Ilich Tchaikovsky, English National Ballet, London, London Coliseum.

Fokine (1911), *Petrushka*, composed by Igor Stravinsky, Ballets Russes, Paris, Théâtre du Châtelet.

Forsythe, William (1987), *In the Middle Somewhat Elevated*, composed by Thom Willems, Paris Opera Ballet, Paris, Opera Garnier.

Hynd, Ronald (1985) (Arthur Saint Léon [1870]), *Coppélia*, composed by Léo Delibes, London Festival Ballet, London, London Coliseum.

MacMillan, Kenneth (1962), *The Rite of Spring*, composed by Igor Stravinsky, Royal Ballet, London, Royal Opera House.

Morris, Mark (1989), *Dido and Aeneas*, composed by Henry Purcell, Mark Morris Dance Group, Brussels, Théâtre Royal de la Monnaie.

Nureyev, Rudolf (1977), *Romeo and Juliet*, composed by Sergei Prokofiev, London Festival Ballet, London, London Coliseum.

Petipa, Marius (1890) (with additions by Kenneth MacMillan [1986]), *The Sleeping Beauty*, composed by Peter Ilich Tchaikovsky, American Ballet Theatre, New York, Kennedy Center Opera House.

—— (1899) (Perrot Jules [1858]), *Le Corsaire*, composed by Adolphe Adam, Imperial Ballet, St Petersburg, Imperial Mariinsky Theatre.

Petit, Roland (1946), *Le Jeune Homme et la Mort*, composed by Johann Sebastian Bach, Ballets des Champs Elysées, Paris, Théâtre des Champs-Élysées.

## Unpublished sources

Anon. 1 (2010), diary.

Canavan, Rachel (2013), questionnaire from author, 29 September.

Dorothy S (2013), diary.

Duff, Joanne (2013), questionnaire from author, 22 February.

Giling, Martin W.L. (2015), 'The Dancer: A Hidden Strength', unpublished poem given by Giling with permission to publish.

Jeffrey, Erica Rose (2016), email correspondence, 9 March.

Jeremy A (2013), diary.

Jim S (2013), diary.

Josephine DG (2013), diary.

Leatherdale, Anna (2013), questionnaire from author, 24 January.

McDonald, Jane (2015), email correspondence with author, 7 April.

Michael B (2011), diary.

Pat K (2011), diary.

Renée A (2014), email correspondence with author, 18 November.

Risch, Roberta (2015), email correspondence with author, 2 April.

Sue (2014), diary.

Sue C (2013), diary.

Taylor, Bob (2013), email correspondence with author, 20 August.

Tham, Hugo (2017), email correspondence with author, 30 October.

## Interviews and conversations

Alan F (2013), in conversation with author, English National Ballet, London, 19 October.

Carroll F (2012a), interview with author, interviewee's home, London, 13 March.

—— (2012b), interview with author, English National Ballet, London, 16 January.

—— (2013), interview with author, The Coliseum, London, 17 January.

Charlotte J (2013), interview with research team member, interviewee's home, London, 8 July.

Christine B (2012), interview with author, English National Ballet, London, 16 January.

Clare N (2010), interview with author, English National Ballet, London, 2 November.

Coldicott, Gemma (2010), interview with author, Purley United Reformed Church, Purley, 5 July.

Derbyshire-Fox, Fleur (2013), interview with author, Virgin Trains, Liverpool, London, 2 February.

Desi B (2013), interview with research team member, interviewee's home, London 4 July.

Dickie, Ann (2010), interview with author, Queen Elizabeth Hall, London, 28 August.

Dorothea (2012), interview with author, interviewee's home, London, 19 October.

Eddie N (2012), interview with author, English National Ballet, London, 5 January.

Ephgrave, Nick (2010), interview with author, National Theatre, London, 15 July.

Fogg, Amanda (2010), interview with author, Weymouth, 8 July.

Godder, Yasmeen (2015), in plenary session of Störung/Hafraah Winter Conversations, Theatre Freiburg, Freiburg, 19 December.

Greenwood, Andrew (2014a), Skype interview with author, 1 August.

—— (2014b), Dance for Parkinson's forum, Bassano del Grappa, 22 August.

Heinz, Herb (2015), FaceTime interview with author, 7 April.

Helena L (2014), interview with author, Merseyside Dance Initiative, Liverpool, 6 February.

Jane D'A (2010), interview with author, interviewee's home, London, 12 November.

—— (2011), interview with author, interviewee's home, London, 22 February.

Jeffery, Erica Rose (2015), Skype interview with author, 4 February.

John H (2012), interview with author, interviewee's home, London, 20 January.

Leonora (2011), interview with author, Mark Morris Dance Center, New York, 17 May.

Leventhal, David (2010), telephone interview with author, 20 July.

Margaret P (2013), interview with author, English National Ballet, London, 19 October.

Mary C (2011), interview with author, interviewee's home, London, 19 February.

Mike A (2011), interview with author, interviewee's home, London, 25 February.

Nichols, Eva (2010), telephone interview with author, 29 September.

Pat C (2012), interview with author, interviewee's home, London, 9 March.

Pat C and Jane D'A (2013), interview with author, The Coliseum, London, 17 January.

Pat K (2010), interview with author, English National Ballet, London, 2 November.

—— (2011), interview with author, English National Ballet, London, 19 February.

—— (2013), interview with research team member, English National Ballet, London, 13 July.

Paul M (2013), interview with research team member, interviewee's home, London, 10 July.

Paul Q (2012), interview with author, English National Ballet, London, 10 March.

Pawar, Hrishikesh (2015), Skype interview with author,16 July.

Ray P (2012a), interview with author, interviewee's home, London, 17 February.

—— (2012b), interview with author, interviewee's home, London, 19 October.

Robert B (2013), interview with author, English National Ballet, London, 19 October.

Roy K (2010), interview with author, English National Ballet, London, 2 November.

—— (2011), interview with author, English National Ballet, London, 19 February.

Sarah W (2016), interview with author, Wimbledon Club, London, 15 February.

Singh, Vonita (2014), Skype interview with author, 17 November.

Vlemmix, Marc (2014), Dance for Parkinson's forum, Bassano del Grappa, 22 August.

—— (2017), in conversation, Dance for Health, Rotterdam, 21 August.

Westheimer, Olie (2010), interview with author, National Theatre, London, 16 July.

—— (2011), interview with author, New York, 17 May.

Zofia (2012), interview with author, interviewee's home, London, 13 January.

## Discussion groups

Discussion group (2013a), English National Ballet Dance for Parkinson's Oxford group, The Old Fire Station, Oxford, 9 March.

—— (2013b), English National Ballet Dance for Parkinson's Oxford group, The Old Fire Station, Oxford, 18 March.

—— (2013c), English National Ballet Dance for Parkinson's Oxford group, The Old Fire Station, Oxford, 6 April.

—— (2014a), English National Ballet Dance for Parkinson's London group, English National Ballet, London, 22 March.

—— (2014b), English National Ballet Dance for Parkinson's London group, English National Ballet, London, 22 May.

—— (2014c), English National Ballet Dance for Parkinson's London group, English National Ballet, London, 21 June.

—— (2014d), English National Ballet Dance for Parkinson's London group, English National Ballet, London, 12 July.

—— (2015), English National Ballet Dance for Parkinson's Ipswich group, DanceEast, London, 22 April.

# Index

Figures are denoted by the use of *italics* and notes by the use of 'n' after the page number.